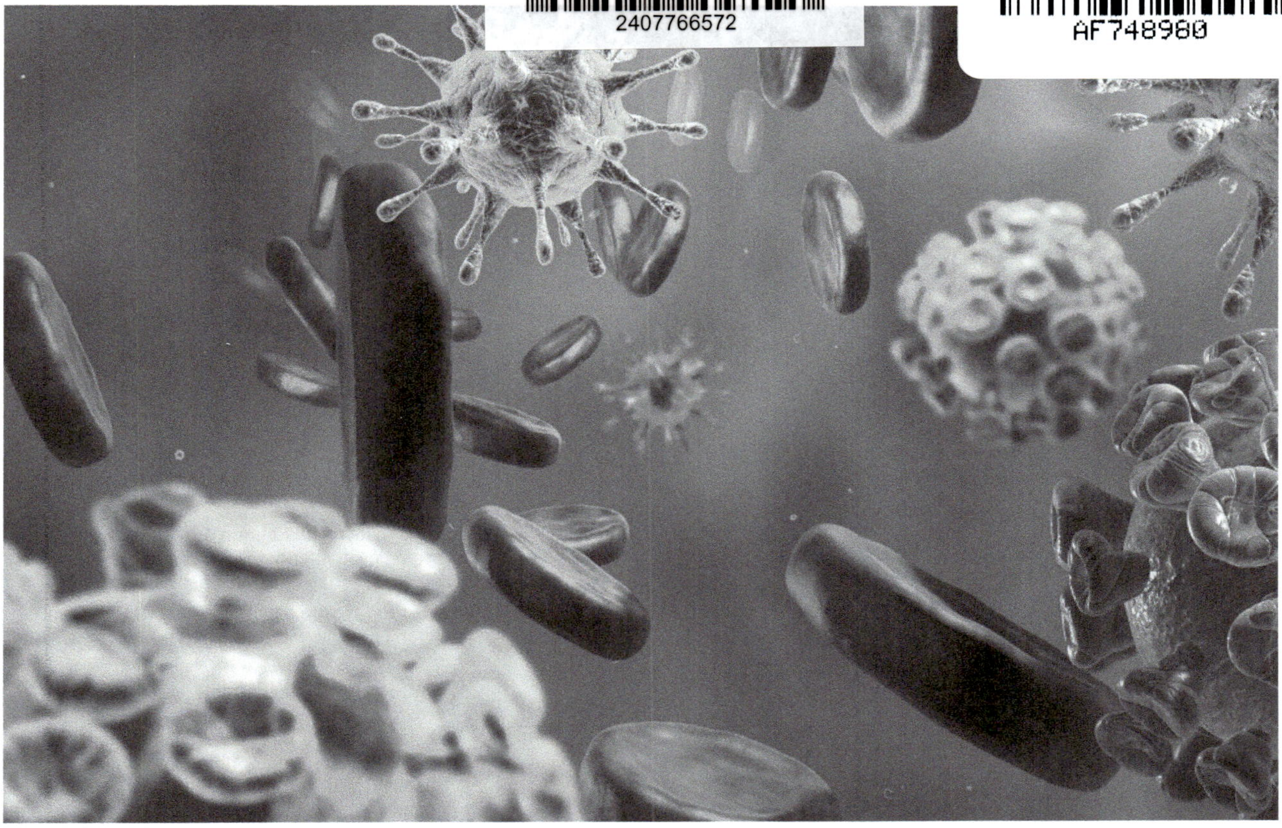

BMJ Easily Missed?:

Cancer, infection and inflammation

Edited by
Professor Anthony Harnden &
Dr Richard Lehman

BPP
UNIVERSITY
SCHOOL OF HEALTH

BPP UNIVERSITY SCHOOL OF HEALTH BMJ

First edition January 2016

ISBN 9781 4727 3896 7
eISBN 9781 4727 3936 0
eISBN 9781 4727 3940 7

British Library Cataloguing-in-Publication Data
A catalogue record for this book is available from the British Library

Published by
BPP Learning Media Ltd
BPP House, Aldine Place
London W12 8AA

www.bpp.com/health

Printed in the United Kingdom by
CPI Antony Rowe

Bumper's Farm,
Chippenham,
Wiltshire
SN14 6LH

Your learning materials, published by BPP Learning Media Ltd, are printed on paper sourced from sustainable, managed forests.

The content of this publication contains articles from The BMJ which have been selected, collated and published by BPP Learning Media under a licence.

About the publisher

BPP Learning Media is dedicated to supporting aspiring professionals with top quality learning material. BPP Learning Media's commitment to success is shown by our record of quality, innovation and market leadership in paper-based and e-learning materials. BPP Learning Media's study materials are written by professionally-qualified specialists who know from personal experience the importance of top quality materials for success.

About The BMJ

The BMJ (formerly the British Medical Journal) in print has a long history and has been published without interruption since 1840. The BMJ's vision is to be the world's most influential and widely read medical journal. Our mission is to lead the debate on health and to engage, inform, and stimulate doctors, researchers, and other health professionals in ways that will improve outcomes for patients. We aim to help doctors to make better decisions. BMJ, the company, advances healthcare worldwide by sharing knowledge and expertise to improve experiences, outcomes and value.

Contents

About the editors

Professor Anthony Harnden is an academic general practitioner at the University of Oxford who has worked five clinical sessions as a partner in general practice in Wheatley, Oxfordshire for more than 25 years. He has published original research papers in general practice related topics, with a focus on children. Professor Harnden is a Deputy Chairman of the Joint Committee of Vaccination and Immunisation (JCVI) and has been responsible for advising the UK government on vaccine policy since 2006. He was the primary care lead for the UK Confidential Enquiry into Child Deaths (2004-8), chaired a group to write a national Royal College of General Practitioners Child Health Strategy (2010-15) and developed the successful series 'Easily Missed?' in The BMJ (2009-).

Dr Richard Lehman is Senior Advisory Fellow in General Practice at the UK Cochrane Centre. He was a full-time general practitioner in Banbury for 32 years. For the last 17 years he has also written a weekly summary of the principal medical journals which is posted on The BMJ website. After retirement from UK general practice in 2010 he has worked on studies of the patient experience, and has spent a year at Yale working with the Yale University Open Data Access (YODA) project and remains a consultant to the group. His main interest is in ways to develop better informed dialogue with patients and he is on the steering committees of the NICE shared decision making initiative and Academy of Medical Royal Colleges Choosing Wisely group.

Foreword

Every clinician misses diagnoses: it's a natural consequence of being human. I am still humbled and upset by missing a cervical cancer many years ago in a 26 year old woman, who died as a consequence. My practice wasn't sloppy – but I could have done things differently leading to the diagnosis emerging much earlier. This brief vignette is a classical 'teaching by anecdote' (and unpopular with educationalists) though perhaps one reader will have a young woman with intermenstrual bleeding consult this week and use this story to identify the cancer. Tell me if you do so, and I'll feel ever so slightly better.

Why do missed diagnoses occur? They arise in two broad areas. The first is where the clinician never thinks of the disorder, or has never even heard of it. At our regular practice meeting of problem cases, I suggested hypokalaemic periodic paralysis as the unifying diagnosis for a supermarket checkout girl who kept dropping things at the till. I was wrong of course, but the other clinicians had never even heard of the condition. Even if we have heard of the disease, it simply may not occur to us; several chapters here are of diseases we would get right in an MCQ but not consider in real life. Who thinks of brucellosis? Or Kawasaki disease, or carcinoid? One newly appointed consultant told me his plan to establish a reputation as a diagnostician was to make as many obscure diagnoses as possible in his early years, saying 'no one will remember when I'm wrong: they won't forget when I'm right'. That wouldn't work in primary care, of course (hypokalaemic period paralysis notwithstanding....).

The second main area in which we miss diagnoses is when we consider them, but decide choose not to investigate because the chance that the patient actually harbours the possible disease is too low. This is sensible clinical behaviour, in that most uninvestigated patients don't have the disease. But some do, and they pay a price. Several of the conditions here are like this: endometriosis, appendicitis, and whooping cough, for example. Delay in such diagnoses causes additional suffering – or worse.

All frontline doctors need to foster a sense of spotting the 'patient who is ill'. This is particularly crucial in infections, especially the rarer ones like HIV, streptococcal disease, malaria and endocarditis. This 'intuition' is a mix of experience and reading. Even better is to add discussion to this mixture: the topics covered here would make splendid teaching points at your practice or hospital clinical meetings (you do have them, don't you).

One diagnostic aphorism I learned early remains useful: for mystery conditions like 'pyrexia of unknown origin' or 'raised inflammatory markers' is that the diagnosis will fall into one of three groups: cancer, infection or inflammation. This book is the first time that I've seen this grouping formalised: read it, discuss it and use it.

Willie Hamilton, MD, FRCP, FRCGP, professor of primary care diagnostics, University of Exeter.

Introduction to Easily Missed series

Patients consult doctors with the expectation of an accurate diagnosis and advice on treatment. But in primary care, patients often present with undifferentiated symptoms without an immediately apparent diagnosis. For most conditions this doesn't matter because the symptoms either resolve or become worse in such a way that the patient returns before any harm is done. In consultations, general practitioners work by using the probability that the collection of presenting symptoms reflects a specific diagnosis. A combination of knowledge, clinical experience, and sound judgment ensures that they usually get it right.

The BMJ series "Easily Missed?" has raised awareness among general practitioners of conditions that are under-recognised in primary care at first presentation. The series has included a wide range of conditions, including some that are common but under-diagnosed and others that are uncommon but so serious that they need to be thought of whenever there is any possibility of their existence.

The articles are short and focused on diagnosis at presentation rather than treatment. The conditions described fulfil four key criteria. Firstly, there is evidence that the condition is commoner than most general practitioners realise or is often missed at first presentation. Secondly, the condition is sufficiently common that the average full time general practitioner in the UK will encounter it at least once a year, or else be so serious that delayed diagnosis is likely to worsen prognosis substantially. Thirdly, the condition has easily defined diagnostic features or diagnostic tests with known predictive characteristics. Fourthly, and most importantly, timely recognition will benefit the patient.

Judging from online access, the series has proved popular amongst readers of The BMJ. We hope that many patients have received early and insightful diagnoses as a result. The series would not have been possible without the dedication, hard work and wisdom of our in house editor, Dr Mabel Chew. She has been a delight to work with and we are very grateful for all her efforts.

Osler said "Medicine is a science of uncertainty and an art of probability." Although uncertainty will always be with us in primary care, the series might teach us more about the art of probability.

Anthony Harnden and Richard Lehman

Colorectal cancer

William Hamilton, professor of primary care diagnostics[1],
Mark G Coleman, director and consultant surgeon[2],
Greg Rubin, professor of general practice and primary care[3]

[1]University of Exeter, Veysey Building, Exeter EX2 4SG, UK

[2]Lapco National Training Programme in Laparoscopic Colorectal Surgery, Derriford Hospital, Plymouth, UK

[3]Durham University, Wolfson Research Institute, Stockton on Tees, UK

Correspondence to: W Hamilton w.hamilton@exeter.ac.uk

Cite as: *BMJ* 2013;346:f3172

DOI: 10.1136/bmj.f3172

www.bmj.com/content/346/bmj.f3172

A 72 year old recently widowed man presents to his general practitioner with vague symptoms, including fatigue. Nothing is found on examination, but his haemoglobin concentration is 114 g/L (range 140-180 g/L) with a hypochromic, normocytic picture and serum ferritin 75 ng/mL (30-336 ng/mL). As his diet has been poor since his wife died, he was treated with ferrous sulphate, which was associated with a small improvement in his fatigue and haemoglobin level. Six months later he presented with intestinal obstruction, which was subsequently found to be due to a carcinoma of the colon.

Surgically, the colon and rectum are distinct, but for the purposes of this diagnostic article, they have been merged.

Why is colorectal cancer missed?

Many colorectal cancers are diagnosed easily and quickly and times to diagnosis (generally measured as the diagnostic interval from first presentation to primary care up to diagnosis) are less than three months—particularly for patients whose clinical features meet the referral guidelines of the National Institute for Health and Clinical Excellence for suspected cancer.[4] Symptoms include diarrhoea or rectal bleeding for six weeks in patients aged more than 60, or for patients older than 40 if both symptoms are present; rectal or abdominal masses or iron deficiency anaemia with haemoglobin concentrations less than 110 g/L in men and less than 100 g/L in women. However, about half of patients do not meet this guidance and have longer diagnostic intervals.[5] Mortality from colorectal cancer is strongly related to the first symptom, with mildly anaemic patients having the worst prognosis; adjusted proportional hazard ratio compared with all patients with colorectal cancer of 1.9 (95% confidence interval 1.1 to 2.7).[6] Audits from several countries suggest that about a third of patients experience diagnostic delays, with anaemia, rectal bleeding, and abdominal pain being the most usual missed opportunities.[7 8 9] These three symptoms are common in primary care, with alternative diagnoses to cancer more likely. Furthermore, NICE guidance recommends urgent investigation only for pronounced iron deficiency anaemia (haemoglobin <110 g/L in men, and <100 g/L in women) or for persistent rectal bleeding (six weeks, unless accompanied by diarrhoea).[4] Additionally, the possibility of cancer may be dismissed in patients with rectal bleeding and haemorrhoids.

Why does this matter?

A complex J-shaped relation exists between the diagnostic interval and mortality.[10] The best prognosis is for patients with an interval of around one month, probably reflecting the timely diagnosis of non-emergency patients. The high mortality with shorter intervals

KEY POINTS

- Patients with mild anaemia can still have colorectal cancer, even if their haemoglobin level is above the threshold recommended by NICE for urgent investigation
- In people aged over 60, women with a haemoglobin concentration ≤110 g/L and men ≤120 g/L and iron deficiency are worth investigating for cancer
- Patients with a new diagnosis of irritable bowel syndrome should have their response to treatment monitored in case of misdiagnosis
- Doctors who record "change in bowel habit" rather than diarrhoea or constipation are potentially thinking of colorectal cancer and further investigations should be considered

probably represents obviously ill patients with an inherently poor prognosis (including emergency admissions). The prognosis steadily worsens with increasing intervals thereafter. Expedited diagnosis may allow identification at an earlier stage, or may obviate emergency admission.

How is colorectal cancer diagnosed?

The rest of this article assumes patients who meet current NICE guidance are investigated, and concentrates on presentations that do not meet NICE guidelines.[4] It does not concern factors before presentation to medical care: there can be major delays from patients not recognising that their symptoms are important.[11] We found no literature suggesting that colorectal cancers in patients under 40 present differently from those in older patients. Similarly, we found no primary care study of colorectal cancer symptoms in patients with inflammatory bowel disease.

Anaemia

Around a third of patients with colorectal cancer in a hospital case series had anaemia but of insufficient severity to meet current NICE guidance, as in our hypothetical case.[12] For those meeting the guidance, the estimated risk of cancer in a large UK case-control study was 13.3% for men and 7.7% for women.[13] The most common measure of iron stores is serum ferritin level, with values below 44.9-67.4 pmol/L (20-30 ng/mL) being regarded as abnormal (individual laboratories have differing ranges). However, in anaemic patients investigated by colonoscopy, those with ferritin levels below 112.4 pmol/L and 112.4-222.5 pmol/L had a similar risk of cancer.[14] Together, this suggests that current guidance is too restrictive. In men aged more than 60 with iron deficiency anaemia, the risk of cancer with a haemoglobin concentration of 110-119 g/L is over 4%; even haemoglobin values of 120-129 g/L represent risks of 3.9% in the 70-79 year age group.[13] The values for women reflect their lower normal haemoglobin range: even so, the risk of cancer in women with haemoglobin concentrations of 110-119 g/L is more than 2.4%. Raising the haemoglobin threshold to allow investigation at such levels would require more colonoscopies but would be in keeping with the threshold risk values used by NICE for other colorectal cancer symptom patterns.[4]

Abdominal pain

Abdominal pain is the most typical symptom of colorectal cancer (alongside rectal bleeding) but it has a low positive predictive value for colorectal cancer of 1.1%, although this increases to 3.0% if abdominal pain is reported again to primary care.[15] When other symptoms, such as diarrhoea or loss of weight, are present, the risk is higher, although rarely above 3%.[15] Few patients with abdominal pain are investigated for possible colorectal cancer at their first presentation. One classic misdiagnosis is irritable bowel syndrome. There is no causative association between irritable bowel syndrome and colorectal cancer; however, around 1% of patients with an initial diagnosis of irritable bowel syndrome prove to have colorectal cancer.[16] All patients with a new diagnosis of irritable bowel syndrome warrant clinical review to confirm that their symptoms are stable and responding to management (diagnostic safety netting). Some guidelines, although not those from NICE, recommend that patients over 50 with new onset irritable bowel syndrome should undergo colonoscopy.

Change in bowel habit and rectal bleeding

Change in bowel habit is a medical term, unused by patients. It is not the same as diarrhoea or constipation, and the risk of cancer is considerably higher when general practitioners' record "change of bowel habit" (3-4% in men aged >60) than when they record diarrhoea (0.9-1.3%) or constipation (0.8%), in the same age group.[17] The most plausible explanation is that when doctors record change in bowel habit they have included other factors in their assessment and deem the total risk to be higher. Arguably, all such patients warrant investigation.

SEARCH STRATEGY

WH and colleagues recently performed a systematic review of primary care symptoms of colorectal cancer.[1] This was supplemented by specific searches on missed or delayed diagnoses, plus searches on young people, irritable bowel syndrome, and inflammatory bowel disease. No randomised controlled trials have been reported on the selection of patients for investigation, so most of the quoted studies are large cohort studies, often using national primary care databases. Cited studies can be assumed to be of this nature unless specifically stated otherwise.

HOW COMMON IS COLORECTAL CANCER?

- Colorectal cancer is the third most prevalent cancer in the United Kingdom, the incidence increasing with age, and it is slightly more common in men
- More than 41 000 new cases of colorectal cancer are diagnosed annually in the United Kingdom, with the median age at diagnosis 72 years, although 6% occur below the age of 40[2]
- Screening identifies a few patients with cancers; the remainder present with symptoms, with around a quarter presenting as an emergency[3]
- A full time general practitioner will have around one patient with a new diagnosis of colorectal cancer each year

Rectal bleeding is a classic symptom of colorectal cancer. In primary care the risk of cancer ranges from 0.5% in women aged less than 60 to 4.5% in men aged more than 80.[17] The risk is higher when diarrhoea is present or when local anal symptoms such as pain, soreness, and itch are absent.[18] A similar pattern of higher risk with increasing age, multiple symptoms, and absent perianal symptoms is seen in the referred population.[19] The Association of Coloproctologists of Great Britain and Ireland have developed a bowel symptom checker for the public and for primary care (www.haveigotbowelcancer.com).

How is colorectal cancer investigated?

Complete examination of the large bowel by colonoscopy after full bowel preparation remains the standard investigation for patients suspected of having bowel cancer. Where colonoscopy is incomplete (in around 11% of patients),[20] it may be repeated, or computed tomography colonography performed. Computed tomography colonography has a similar identification rate for cancer and polyps to that of colonoscopy, and both are superior to barium enema.[20 21] All the standard investigations have low false negative rates, although persistent symptoms may require reinvestigation.[22]

How is colorectal cancer managed?

National guidance on the management of colorectal cancer was published in November 2011.[23] Surgery, either open or laparoscopic, is the primary treatment. Adjuvant treatments include postoperative chemotherapy in patients with node positive (Dukes' stage C) results, and preoperative radiotherapy, which reduces the risk of local recurrence in rectal cancer. Metastases to the liver or lung may also be resected. Patients presenting with large bowel obstruction can sometimes be decompressed with an endoscopically placed stent, allowing resection later.

We thank Eustacia Hamilton for help with the initial searches.

Contributors: WH performed the initial searches and drafted the first version of the article. All three authors revised the article, adding additional references. WH is the guarantor.

Competing interests. All authors have completed the ICMJE uniform disclosure form at www.icmje.org/coi_disclosure.pdf (available on request from the corresponding author) and declare: WH has received several research grants for studies on cancer diagnosis, including one from Colonix, a commercial firm. He is the clinical lead for the current revision of the NICE 2005 guidance. His contribution to this article is in a personal capacity and is not to be interpreted as representing the view of the Guideline Development Group or of NICE itself. He has received travel support to give lectures and attend conferences, plus occasional modest speaker's fees, from conference organisers in the charitable and educational sector, though none from commercial sources. MGC is the national lead clinician for the Lapco National Training Programme in Laparoscopic Colorectal Surgery. He is the chairman of external affairs for the Association of Coloproctologists of Great Britain and Ireland and a national peer review advisor for the hepatopancreaticobiliary cancer peer review group. His contribution to this article is in a personal capacity. He has received travel support to give lectures and attend conferences, plus fees, from conference organisers in the educational sector, and some from commercial sources to lecture abroad on laparoscopic colorectal surgery from Olympus, Johnson & Johnson and Covidien. GR is the Royal College of General Practitioners clinical lead for cancer, a post part funded by Cancer Research UK. He has received support for travel and conference attendance, and payment for advisory services from Lilly, Almirall, and Warner Chilcott. His contribution to this article is in a personal capacity. All authors are members of the Bowel Cancer UK Medical Advisory Board. No other relationships or activities that could appear to have influenced the submitted work.

Provenance and peer review: Commissioned; externally peer reviewed.

Patient consent not required (patient anonymised, dead, or hypothetical).

1 Astin M, Griffin T, Neal RD, Rose P, Hamilton W. The diagnostic value of symptoms for colorectal cancer in primary care: a systematic review. *Br J Gen Pract* 2011;61:e231-43.
2 Cancer Research UK. CancerStats key facts: bowel cancer. Cancer Research UK, 2012.
3 Elliss-Brookes L, McPhail S, Ives A, Greenslade M, Shelton J, Hiom S, et al. Routes to diagnosis for cancer—determining the patient journey using multiple routine data sets. *Br J Cancer* 201;107:1220-6.
4 National Institute for Health and Clinical Excellence. Referral guidelines for suspected cancer. NICE, 2005.
5 Hamilton W. Cancer diagnosis in primary care. *Br J Gen Pract* 2010;60:121-8.
6 Stapley S, Peters TJ, Sharp D, Hamilton W. The mortality of colorectal cancer in relation to the initial symptom and to the duration of symptoms: a cohort study in primary care. *Br J Cancer* 2006;95:1321-5.
7 Singh H, Daci K, Petersen LA, Collins C, Petersen NJ, Shethia A, et al. Missed opportunities to initiate endoscopic evaluation for colorectal cancer diagnosis. *Am J Gastroenterol* 2009;104:2543-54.
8 Domínguez-Ayala M, Díez-Vallejo J, Comas-Fuentes A. Missed opportunities in early diagnosis of symptomatic colorectal cancer. *Rev Esp Enfirm Dig* 2012;104:343-9.
9 Damery S, Ryan R, Wilson S, Ismail T, Hobbs R, On behalf of the Improving Colorectal Outcomes Group. Iron deficiency anaemia and delayed diagnosis of colorectal cancer: a retrospective cohort study. *Colorectal Dis* 2011;13:e53-60.
10 Torring M, Frydenberg M, Hansen R, Olesen F, Hamilton W, Vedsted P. Time to diagnosis and mortality in colorectal cancer: a cohort study in primary care. *Br J Cancer* 2011;104:934-40.
11 Thompson MR, Heath I, Swarbrick ET, Faulds Wood L, Ellis BG. Earlier diagnosis and treatment of symptomatic bowel cancer: can it be achieved and how much will it improve survival? *Colorectal Dis* 2011;13:6-16.
12 Masson S, Chinn DJ, Tabaqchali MA, Waddup G, Dwarakanath AD. Is anaemia relevant in the referral and diagnosis of colorectal cancer? *Colorectal Dis* 2007;9:736-9.
13 Hamilton W, Lancashire R, Sharp D, Peters TJ, Cheng K, Marshall T. The importance of anaemia in diagnosing colorectal cancer: a case-control study using electronic primary care records. *Br J Cancer* 2008;98:323-7.
14 Sawhney MS, Lipato T, Nelson DB, Lederle FA, Rector TS, Bond JH. Should patients with anemia and low normal or normal serum ferritin undergo colonoscopy? *Am J Gastroenterol* 2007;102:82-8.
15 Hamilton W, Round A, Sharp D, Peters T. Clinical features of colorectal cancer before diagnosis: a population-based case-control study. *Br J Cancer* 2005;93:399-405.
16 García Rodríguez L, Ruigómez A, Wallander M, Johansson S, Olbe L. Detection of colorectal tumor and inflammatory bowel disease during follow-up of patients with initial diagnosis of irritable bowel syndrome. *Scand J Gastroenterol* 2000:35:306-11.
17 Hamilton W, Lancashire R, Sharp D, Peters TJ, Cheng KK, Marshall T. The risk of colorectal cancer with symptoms at different ages and between the sexes: a case-control study. *BMC Med* 2009;7:17.
18 Ellis BG, Thompson M. Factors identifying higher risk rectal bleeding in general practice. *Br J Gen Pract* 2005;55:949-55.
19 Thompson MR, Perera R, Senapati A, Dodds S. Predictive value of common symptom combinations in diagnosing colorectal cancer. *Br J Surg* 2007;94:1260-5.
20 Atkin W, Dadswell E, Wooldrage K, Kralj-Hans I, von Wagner C, Edwards R, et al. Computed tomographic colonography versus colonoscopy for investigation of patients with symptoms suggestive of colorectal cancer (SIGGAR): a multicentre randomised trial. *Lancet* 2013; published online 14 Feb.
21 Halligan S, Wooldrage K, Dadswell E, Kralj-Hans I, von Wagner C, Edwards R, et al. Computed tomographic colonography versus barium enema for diagnosis of colorectal cancer or large polyps in symptomatic patients (SIGGAR): a multicentre randomised trial. *Lancet* 2013; published online 14 Feb.
22 Johnson CD, Chen M-H, Toledano AY, Heiken JP, Dachman A, Kuo MD, et al. Accuracy of CT colonography for detection of large adenomas and cancers. *N Engl J Med* 2008;359:1207-17.
23 National Institute for Health and Clinical Excellence. Colorectal cancer: the diagnosis and management of colorectal cancer: CG131. NICE, 2011.

Lung cancer

Richard D Neal, professor of primary care medicine[1],
William Hamilton, professor of primary care diagnostics[2],
Trevor K Rogers, consultant respiratory physician[3]

[1]North Wales Centre for Primary Care Research, Bangor University, Wrexham LL13 7YP, UK

[2]Department of Primary Care Diagnostics, University of Exeter Medical School, Exeter, UK

[3]Doncaster Royal Infirmary, Doncaster and Bassetlaw NHS Foundation Trust, Doncaster, UK

Correspondence to: R D Neal r.neal@bangor.ac.uk

Cite this as: *BMJ* 2014;349:g6560

DOI: 10.1136/bmj.g6560

www.bmj.com/content/349/bmj.g6560

A 65 year old recent ex-smoker with a 20 pack year history and chronic obstructive pulmonary disease (COPD) consults his general practitioner because of worse chest symptoms over the past three weeks, with increasing breathlessness and production of green sputum, and a feeling of being "off colour." Similar previous spells have been treated with antibiotics and steroids to good effect. On examination his temperature is normal, his heart rate is 88 beats/min, respiratory rate is 16 breaths/min, and oxygen saturation is 94% on air. He has tobacco stained fingers but no clubbing or evidence of weight loss. Scattered crackles and wheezes are found on auscultation of the lungs. After treatment with antibiotics and steroids he feels no better, and after two further consultations he is referred for chest radiography, which is reported as showing a lesion suspicious of lung cancer.

Lung cancer

Lung cancer refers to primary tumours of the lung and is initially classified histologically as small cell lung cancer (SCLC) or non-small cell lung cancer (NSCLC) because these two types behave very differently. The main forms of NSCLC are squamous, adenocarcinoma, and neuroendocrine large cell cancers. This subdivision has become more important with the advent of tailored chemotherapy for advanced disease based on the subtype of NSCLC and biological drugs for some adenocarcinomas. These include tyrosine kinase inhibitors in tumours with sensitising mutations in the epidermal growth factor receptor and, even more recently, anaplastic lymphoma kinase inhibitors.

Why is it missed?

Lung cancer is harder to diagnose than most other cancers so the diagnosis is often delayed. There is evidence from recent well conducted cohort studies that:

- A third of patients consulted their GP about the health problem caused by cancer three or more times before referral (third highest of the 18 cancers reported)[3]
- The median diagnostic interval (time from first presentation to diagnosis) is 112 days (interquartile range 45-251)—the second highest of the 15 cancers reported[4]
- The median primary care interval (time from first presentation to referral) is 14 days (3-40) (only myeloma is higher) and increases with increasing numbers of pre-referral consultations[3]
- Thirty nine per cent of lung cancers present as an emergency (a marker for poor outcomes)—only cancers of the brain and pancreas are higher.[5]

THE BOTTOM LINE

- Suspect lung cancer in all at-risk patients (age, smoking, chronic obstructive pulmonary disease) with a new respiratory symptom, or atypical non-respiratory symptom, even if they appear otherwise well
- Consider lung cancer in non-smokers with suspicious symptoms, especially haemoptysis and multiple symptoms
- Chest radiography is cheap, easy, widely available, and relatively harm free, but can be falsely negative. Have a low threshold for repeating or referring for specialist opinion (or considering computed tomography if available) if there are diagnostic suspicions
- Aim to diagnose patients as quickly as possible to optimise the chance of cure and active anti-cancer treatment

The diagnosis may be initially missed because of lack of a clear "symptom signature,"[6] symptomatic "noise" resulting from COPD and other comorbidities,[7 8] chest radiographs being reported as normal or benign findings,[9] presentation with non-respiratory or atypical symptoms, or patient mediated factors (such as delay in re-presenting or declining earlier referral).

Why does this matter?

Overall, lung cancer has a poor prognosis. Longer diagnostic intervals are associated with increased mortality,[10] with fewer patients being amenable to curative treatments. There may also be morbidity and quality of life benefits from more timely diagnosis, although this has not been proved. Certainly, late diagnosis creates enormous challenges for patients and their families in coming to terms with the diagnosis, planning for their changed circumstances, and resolving their affairs. It is not unusual for patients to present for the first time as a medical emergency and then to die in hospital.[5]

How is it diagnosed?

Chest radiography is the main investigation that leads to diagnosis. In about 10% of patients subsequently diagnosed with lung cancer, the initial radiograph is reported as normal, and indeterminate abnormalities are found in a further 13%.[9] Computed tomography is used largely in specialist practice, either when the radiograph is negative but cancer is still suspected or when the radiograph shows an abnormality. Further invasive tests are then undertaken to provide a tissue diagnosis. Thus, identification in primary care, where most patients initially present,[11] generally hinges on identifying features that prompt a chest radiograph or that require specialist investigation even if the radiograph is normal, such as persistent haemoptysis in an older smoker. Thus, we concentrate on features that may prompt a request for chest radiography.

A recent systematic review collated five primary care reports of lung cancer symptoms.[6] Positive predictive values (PPVs, which express the risk of cancer numerically) of symptoms were: cough 0.4% in two studies, weight loss 1.1% and 6.1% in two studies, and appetite loss 0.9% and 4.7% in two studies. The classic feature of lung cancer—haemoptysis—had a PPV of 2.4-7.5%. However, only a minority of primary care patients with lung cancer report haemoptysis.[11] PPVs increase with age, current smoking, and multiple or persistent symptoms.[11 12 13]

Three algorithms for the diagnosis of lung cancer have been created: the simplest, a risk assessment tool, offers PPVs for pairs of symptoms or for repeated symptoms, stratified into smokers and non-smokers. In a before and after study, use of the tool was accompanied by increased requests for chest radiography and lung cancer diagnosis, including early stage cancers.[14] Q-cancer and a second algorithm are multivariable equations that incorporate data on risk factors as well as symptoms.[12 13] Their theoretical performance is good, but no reports of actual performance are available. Risk assessment tools and Q-cancer have been incorporated into all UK based primary care clinical software systems and can be programmed to prompt the GP once a lung cancer risk above an agreed threshold has been estimated.

Patients who present with symptoms recommended by the National Institute for Health and Care Excellence (NICE) for investigation have shorter times to diagnosis compared with those without these symptoms.[4 15] This reflects possible alternative diagnoses for the "low risk but not no risk" symptoms, such as cough, plus the atypical presentations, especially with metastases.

How is it managed?

Treatment in the United Kingdom is based on NICE guidance and depends on histological type, disease stage, fitness, performance status, and patient preference.[16] Tissue diagnosis is commonly achieved at bronchoscopy, sometimes using endobronchial ultrasound, or

HOW COMMON IS IT?

- In 2011, there were 43 463 new cases of lung cancer in the United Kingdom, making it the second most common cancer and representing 13% of all new cancers[1]
- The crude incidence rate is 77 cancer cases per 100 000 men in the UK, and 61 per 100 000 women
- In most cases there is a history of smoking, and incidence increases with age
- Patients with chronic obstructive pulmonary disease are about four times more likely to develop lung cancer than those without (1% risk/year)[2]
- Lung cancer accounts for 22% of deaths from cancer in the UK. An average GP will see about one new diagnosis of lung cancer each year

imaging guided needle biopsy. In NSCLC, if the tumour appears localised on the diagnostic computed tomogram, staging positron emission tomography-computed tomography is needed to establish eligibility for curative treatment. When the disease is localised and the patient has adequate physiological reserve, surgery is the treatment of choice. If the tumour is unresectable, radiotherapy is an alternative radical option, provided the disease can be encompassed in a treatment volume. Stereotactic ablative radiotherapy is increasingly available as a curative option in patients with peripheral tumours and borderline fitness. Multimodality treatment may increase cure rates and should be considered in fitter patients. When radical treatment is not possible in NSCLC and functional status is good, chemotherapy can improve life expectancy and symptom control. Highly effective biological agents are now available for the minority of adenocarcinomas that carry specific sensitising mutations.

For localised SCLC, chemoradiotherapy can be given with curative intent, and chemotherapy has prognostic and palliative value in the remaining patients, provided they are fit enough. The substantial majority of patients who present with advanced disease of whatever histological type can benefit from palliative treatments, including radiotherapy and specialist palliative care. However, resection rates are improving,[17] and there are encouraging signs that early diagnostic initiatives, such as the use of risk assessment tools, may have benefit[14]—particularly in reducing the number of emergency admissions.

Contributors: RDN wrote the first draft of most of the paper. WH wrote the first draft of the "How is it diagnosed?" section. TKR wrote the first draft of the "How is it managed?" section. All three authors then revised the paper critically. All authors agree to be accountable for the work. RDN is guarantor.

Competing interests: We have read and understood BMJ policy on declaration of interests and declare the following interests: WH is clinical adviser for the current revision of the NICE 2005 guidance, CG27, on the topic of selection of patients for cancer investigation. His contribution to this article is in a personal capacity, and does not represent the view of the Guideline Development Group, or of NICE itself. RDN sits on two funding boards (Roy Castle Lung Cancer Foundation and the RCGP scientific foundation board) that may fund research into the early diagnosis of lung cancer. RDN and WH hold grants from several bodies (including the National Institute for Health Research, Department of Health, Cancer Research UK, Tenovus, Cancer Research Wales, Betsi Cadwaladr University Health Board, Public Health Wales, and National Institute for Social Care and Health Research) to undertake research into the early diagnosis of cancer. WH has received funding from charities including Macmillan to give lectures and attend conferences.

Provenance and peer review: Commissioned; externally peer reviewed.

Patient consent not required (patient anonymised, dead, or hypothetical).

1 Cancer Research UK. Lung cancer incidence statistics. 2014. www.cancerresearchuk.org/cancer-info/cancerstats/types/lung/incidence/uk-lung-cancer-incidence-statistics.

2 Kiri VA, Soriano J, Visick G, Fabbri L. Recent trends in lung cancer and its association with COPD: an analysis using the UK GP Research Database. *Prim Care Respir J* 2010;19:57-61.

3 Lyratzopoulos G, Abel GA, McPhail S, Neal RD, Rubin GP. Measures of promptness of cancer diagnosis in primary care: secondary analysis of national audit data on patients with 18 common and rarer cancers. *Br J Cancer* 2013;108:686-90.

4 Neal RD, Din NU, Hamilton W, Ukoumunne O, Carter BR, Stapley S, et al. Comparison of cancer diagnostic intervals before and after implementation of NICE guidelines: analysis of data from the UK General Practice Research Database. *Br J Cancer* 2014;110:584-92.

5 Elliss-Brookes L, McPhail S, Ives A, Greenslade M, Shelton J, Hiom S, et al. Routes to diagnosis for cancer—determining the patient journey using multiple routine data sets. *Br J Cancer* 2012;107:1220-6.

6 Shin S, Brindle L, Simon M, George S. A systematic review of symptomatic diagnosis of lung cancer. *Fam Pract* 2014;31:137-48.

7 Mitchell ED, Rubin G, Macleod U. Understanding diagnosis of lung cancer in primary care: qualitative synthesis of significant event audit reports. *Br J Gen Pract* 2013;63:e37-46.

8 Neal RD, Robbé IJ, Lewis M, Williamson I, Hanson J. The complexity and difficulty of diagnosing lung cancer: findings from a national primary care study in Wales. *Primary Health Care Res Development* [forthcoming].

9 Stapley S, Sharp D, Hamilton W. Negative chest X-rays in primary care patients with lung cancer. *Br J Gen Pract* 2006;56:570-3.

10 Tørring ML, Frydenberg M, Hansen RP, Olesen F, Vedsted P. Evidence of increasing mortality with longer diagnostic intervals for five common cancers: a cohort study in primary care. *Eur J Cancer* 2013;49:2187-98.

11 Hamilton W, Peters T, Round A, Sharp D. What are the clinical features of lung cancer before the diagnosis is made? A population based case-control study. *Thorax* 2005;60:1059-65.

12 Hippisley-Cox J, Coupland C. Identifying patients with suspected lung cancer in primary care: derivation and validation of an algorithm. *Br J Gen Pract* 2011;61:e715-23.

13 Iyen-Omofoman B, Tata LJ, Baldwin DR, Smith CJP, Hubbard RB. Using socio-demographic and early clinical features in general practice to identify people with lung cancer earlier. *Thorax* 2013;68:451-9.

14 Hamilton W, Green T, Martins T, Elliott K, Rubin G, Macleod U. Evaluation of risk assessment tools for suspected cancer in general practice: a cohort study. *Br J Gen Pract* 2013;63:e30-6.

15 National Institute of Health and Care Excellence. Referral for suspected cancer. Clinical Guideline 27. 2005. www.nice.org.uk/guidance/cg27.

16 National Institute of Health and Care Excellence. The diagnosis and treatment of lung cancer. Clinical Guideline 121. 2011. www.nice.org.uk/guidance/cg121.

17 Treasure T, Russell C, Morton D, Macbeth F, Utley M. Surgical resection of lung cancer England: more operations but no trials to test their effectiveness. *Thorax* 2012;67:759-61.

Ovarian cancer

William Hamilton, consultant senior lecturer[1],
Usha Menon, professor and consultant gynaecologist[2]

[1]Academic Unit of Primary Health Care, Department of Community Based Medicine, University of Bristol, Bristol BS6 2AA

[2]Academic Gynaecological Oncology, UCL EGA Institute for Women's Health, Maple House, London W1T 7DN

Correspondence to: U Menon u.menon@ucl.ac.uk

Cite this as: *BMJ* 2009;339:b4650

DOI: 10.1136/bmj.b4650

www.bmj.com/content/339/bmj.b4650

Ovarian cancer is the leading cause of death from gynaecological cancer in the United Kingdom. Around 4400 deaths occur each year, and UK mortality figures are worse than comparable European ones.[1]

Why is it missed?

The vagueness and non-specific nature of the symptoms, lack of serious pain or physical disability, and lack of awareness cause women to dismiss the symptoms as being related to normal body changes, such as the menopause, or to stress.[2] The initial symptoms are often suggestive of benign gastrointestinal or urinary conditions, which are also much more common than ovarian cancer. The predominance of gastrointestinal symptoms means that women are often misdiagnosed as having irritable bowel syndrome or gastritis.[3] In women over 50, the new onset of irritable bowel syndrome-like symptoms should raise the possibility of serious disease, including ovarian cancer.

Even if cancer is considered, colorectal cancer is more common, and patients are often sent on the wrong investigative pathway. Current UK referral guidelines recommend urgent investigation only in the presence of abnormal vaginal bleeding or a palpable pelvic mass.[4] Both are uncommon early features. Screening is not available—it is still being evaluated in large randomised controlled trials.

Why does this matter?

Ovarian cancer is staged by the International Federation of Obstetrics and Gynaecology (FIGO) system. Most women present with advanced stage disease (FIGO III and IV), which is associated with a five year survival of 25-30% compared with 80-90% in those diagnosed in early stages (FIGO I or II). The median time to diagnosis is reported as less than three months in 55% of women, but it was more than six months in 26% and more than a year in 11%.[3] Women who ignored their symptoms or presented with gastrointestinal symptoms were significantly more likely to be diagnosed with advanced disease.[3 5]

How is it diagnosed?

Clinical diagnosis

Because the incidence of ovarian cancer is relatively low, positive predictive values for most symptoms are low (table).[6 7] Abdominal distension is usually persistent and progressive, unlike bloating, which most clinicians use to mean intermittent distension. However, women have their own interpretation of these terms, so it is important to clarify what is meant.[8]

KEY POINTS

- Any of the following three symptoms should raise the possibility of ovarian cancer especially if they occur on most days, are persistent, or worsening—persistent pelvic or abdominal pain (or both); increased abdominal size or persistent bloating; and difficulty eating and feeling full quickly. Other symptoms such as urinary symptoms, change in bowel habit, extreme fatigue, or back pain may also occur, with or without those listed above
- In women over 50 years, onset of irritable bowel syndrome-like symptoms should raise the possibility of serious disease, including ovarian cancer
- Perform an abdominal and pelvic examination and request serum CA125 and pelvic ultrasonography if ovarian cancer is suspected, especially in women over 50
- When findings are negative, women should be encouraged to return if symptoms become more frequent or more pronounced

Table 1 Main symptoms of ovarian cancer

Symptom	Frequency reported to GP before diagnosis	Positive predictive value in primary care
Abdominal pain	53%	0.3%
Fatigue	39%	Unknown, but will be small
Abdominal distension	36%	2.5%
Diarrhoea	27%	Unknown, but will be small
Bloating	17%	0.3%
Pelvic pain	16%	Unknown
Increased urinary frequency	14%	0.2%
Abnormal vaginal bleeding	13%	0.5%
Weight loss	10%	Unknown

HOW COMMON IS IT?

- Just under 7000 new diagnoses are made each year in the United Kingdom
- This equates to about one new diagnosis for each full time general practitioner every five years
- About 85% of new cases are diagnosed in women over 50 years

CASE SCENARIO

Susan was 52 when she first noticed symptoms of urinary urgency, then abdominal swelling and intermittent abdominal pain. Because at the time she was tearful and tired as a result of work difficulties, and urinalysis was normal, her general practitioner thought that she was depressed. After several more attendances, however, her abdomen was examined, and a mass was felt on vaginal examination. Rapid investigation, including transvaginal ultrasound and serum CA125, led to surgery and a diagnosis of stage III ovarian cancer.

A symptom index of pelvic or abdominal pain, increased abdominal size or bloating, and difficulty eating or feeling full, when present for more than a year and occurring on more than 12 days a month, had a sensitivity of 56.7% for early stage disease and 79.5% for advanced stage disease. Specificity was 90% for women age over 50 in a US primary care setting and 86.7% for women under 50 years.[9]

In the UK, recent guidance urges doctors to look for ovarian cancer in patients with the above symptoms, especially if they are of recent onset and persistent.[10] A similar awareness campaign is under way in the United States. Abdominal and pelvic examinations are important—almost half of women may have a palpable mass at diagnosis. If the examination is negative, women should be encouraged to return if symptoms become more frequent or pronounced.

Investigations

Serum CA125 and transvaginal ultrasound had a specificity of 95% and 92%, respectively, in a pilot study of symptomatic women over 45 years in primary care.[11] Their sensitivity in symptomatic women in primary care is unknown, so a negative test cannot completely rule out cancer. The preferred investigation is a combination of CA125 and pelvic (ideally transvaginal) ultrasound, which is more sensitive and more specific than either alone in distinguishing benign from malignant adnexal masses.[12] A "risk of malignancy index"—which combines CA125, menopausal status, and transvaginal ultrasound findings—is often used to differentiate malignant ovarian masses from benign ones.[13]

How is it managed?

Surgery is the primary intervention in suspected ovarian cancer, both to obtain histological confirmation and stage as well as first line treatment. In women who have completed their families, this usually means laparotomy with removal of the uterus, fallopian tubes, ovaries, part of the omentum, and any relevant biopsies. If disease is advanced, "debulking" surgery is performed with the aim of leaving behind as little tumour as possible. Increasing evidence points to minimal residual disease being associated with better prognosis. Immediately after surgery, many women are given adjuvant chemotherapy, normally a platinum compound with paclitaxel added on an individual basis.

Contributors: WH wrote the first draft, with revision by UM. Both authors are guarantors.

Competing interests: None declared.

Patient consent not required (patient anonymised, dead, or hypothetical).

Provenance and peer review: Commissioned; externally peer reviewed.

1 Verdecchia A, Francisci S, Brenner H, Gatta G, Micheli A, Mangone L, et al. Recent cancer survival in Europe: a 2000-02 period analysis of EUROCARE-4 data. *Lancet Oncol* 2007;8:784-96.
2 Fitch M, Deane K, Howell D, Gray R. Women's experiences with ovarian cancer: reflections on being diagnosed. *Can Oncol Nurs J* 2002;12:152-68.
3 Goff BA, Mandel L, Muntz HG, Melancon CH. Ovarian carcinoma diagnosis. *Cancer* 2000;89:2068-75.
4 National Institute for Health and Clinical Excellence. *Referral guidelines for suspected cancer*. London: NICE, 2005.
5 Ryerson AB, Eheman C, Burton J, McCall N, Blackman D, Subramanian S, et al. Symptoms, diagnoses, and time to key diagnostic procedures among older US women with ovarian cancer. *Obstet Gynecol* 2007;109:1053-61.
6 Friedman GD, Skilling JS, Udaltsova NV, Smith LH. Early symptoms of ovarian cancer: a case-control study without recall bias. *Fam Pract* 2005;22:548-53.
7 Hamilton W, Peters TJ, Bankhead C, Sharp D. Risk of ovarian cancer in women with symptoms in primary care: population based case-control study. *BMJ* 2009;339:b2998.
8 Bankhead C, Collins C, Stokes-Lampard H, Rose P, Wilson S, Clements A, et al. Identifying symptoms of ovarian cancer: a qualitative and quantitative study. *BJOG* 2008;115:1008-14.
9 Goff BA, Mandel LS, Drescher CW, Urban N, Gough S, Schurman KM, et al. Development of an ovarian cancer symptom index: possibilities for earlier detection. *Cancer* 2007;109:221-7.
10 Department of Health. Ovarian cancer: key messages for health professionals, 2009.
11 Rufford BD, Jacobs IJ, Menon U. Feasibility of screening for ovarian cancer using symptoms as selection criteria. *BJOG* 2007;114:59-64.
12 Myers ER, Bastian LA, Havrilesky LJ, Kulasingam SL, Terplan MS, Cline KE, et al. Management of adnexal mass. *Evid Rep Technol Assess* 2006;130:1-145.
13 Jacobs IJ, Oram D, Fairbanks J, Turner J, Frost C, Grudzinskas J. A risk of malignancy index incorporating CA 125, ultrasound and menopausal status for the accurate preoperative diagnosis of ovarian cancer. *BJOG* 1990;97:922-9.

Pancreatic cancer

Ajith K Siriwardena, professor of hepatobiliary surgery[1,2], Alison M Siriwardena, salaried general practitioner[3]

[1]Regional Hepato-Pancreato-Biliary Unit, Manchester Royal Infirmary, Manchester M13 9WL, UK

[2]University of Manchester, Manchester, UK

[3]Bramhall Park Medical Centre, Stockport, UK

Correspondence to: A K Siriwardena ajith.siriwardena@cmft.nhs.uk

Cite this as: *BMJ* 2014;349:g6385

DOI: 10.1136/bmj.g6385

www.bmj.com/content/349/bmj.g6385

A 74 year old man who had been self medicating with antacids for recurrent indigestion consulted his general practitioner when symptoms persisted for three months. After assessment his GP prescribed a proton pump inhibitor and arranged review in four weeks. Two months later he developed back pain and was prescribed paracetamol with advice about mobilisation. Within four weeks he developed jaundice with dark urine and was admitted to his local hospital. Contrast enhanced computed tomography confirmed a diagnosis of locally advanced, unresectable pancreatic cancer (figure). He received palliative chemotherapy but died five months later.

Pancreatic cancer

More than eight in 10 cases of pancreatic cancer are ductal adenocarcinoma arising from the epithelium of the exocrine pancreas.[1] Obstruction of the lower common bile duct gives rise to the classic presentation of painless obstructive jaundice (dark urine, pale stools, and pruritus owing to hyperbilirubinaemia).[2] Tumours can also arise from the body or tail of the gland, and these are particularly difficult to diagnose because symptoms tend to be a late feature.[3,4]

Surgical resection followed by adjuvant chemotherapy is the optimum treatment, but most patients are unsuitable for surgery because of comorbidity or the tumour being locally advanced or metastatic.[7,8]

Why is it missed?

Pancreatic cancer is easily missed at initial presentation because the early symptoms are non-specific and common. Non-specific symptoms can be categorised as systemic or "local." Systemic features include weight loss and the onset of diabetes or impaired glucose tolerance.[9]Local symptoms include abdominal pain and back pain. Abdominal pain, often epigastric and radiating to the back, is easily mistaken for dyspepsia by patients and doctors. Back pain is also common in pancreatic cancer,[10] possibly because extrapancreatic spread can involve peri-pancreatic neural plexuses. However, back pain is common in the age group most affected by pancreatic cancer, and in the absence of other symptoms or signs is unlikely to raise a suspicion of pancreatic cancer at first presentation.

Jaundice is a relatively late symptom. Typically, the onset of jaundice precipitates consultation and rapid onward referral. Obstruction of the main pancreatic duct can lead to compromise in exocrine function, which can manifest as fat intolerance, steatorrhoea, and weight loss.[10] This clinical picture is a late stage phenomenon, but milder symptoms may be noticeable at an early stage.

THE BOTTOM LINE

- Consider the diagnosis of pancreatic cancer in all patients presenting with painless obstructive jaundice and refer for further assessment
- Consider the diagnosis in patients with persistent non-specific gastrointestinal symptoms combined with recent onset or atypical back pain or recent onset diabetes
- Early referral, assessment, and surgical resection with adjuvant chemotherapy are the mainstays of care for patients with resectable disease, but most patients are not candidates for surgery
- In patients with unresectable disease, direct treatment towards the relief of jaundice, adequate analgesia, establishment of a tissue diagnosis, consideration of chemotherapy, pancreatic exocrine replacement, and appropriate palliative care

Table 1 Algorithm for the diagnosis of pancreatic cancer. Data expressed as adjusted hazard ratios (95% confidence interval)[14]

Factor	Women (95% CI)	Men (95% CI)
Smoking status		
Non-smoker	1	1
Ex-smoker	0.97 (0.77 to 1.23)	1.37 (1.12 to 1.67)
Light smoker	1.53 (1.04 to 2.25)	1.44 (1.03 to 2.03)
Moderate smoker	2.32 (1.74 to 3.10)	1.63 (1.20 to 2.20)
Heavy smoker	2.39 (1.65 to 3.48)	1.88 (1.36 to 2.61)
Medical history		
Type 2 diabetes	2.07 (1.66 to 2.58)	2.11 (1.76 to 2.52)
Chronic pancreatitis	3.15 (1.17 to 8.46)	3.94 (1.93 to 8.01)
Current symptoms and symptoms in preceding year		
Current appetite loss*	3.90 (2.61 to 5.82)	2.46 (1.43 to 4.23)
Current weight loss*	3.27 (2.35 to 4.56)	12.5 (7.84 to 19.9)†
Current abdominal pain*	4.09 (3.46 to 4.84)	5.23 (4.48 to 6.11)
Current abdominal distension*	3.04 (1.68 to 5.50)	NS‡
Current dysphagia*	NS	2.56 (1.60 to 4.10)
Constipation in past year*	NS	1.91 (1.35 to 2.71)

**Compared with person without this characteristic.*
†Interaction term at mean age in men. The model for men also included an interaction between weight loss and the age term. Hazard ratios adjusted for all other terms in the table and for age.
‡NS=not significant.

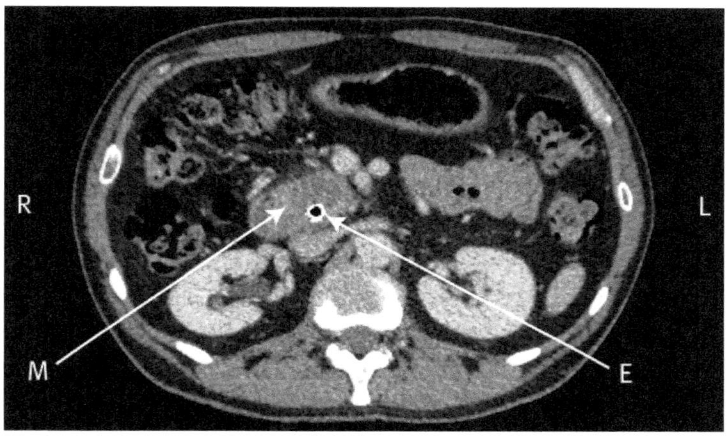

Fig 1 Contrast enhanced computed tomogram of the upper abdomen showing a hypodense (dark) mass (M) in the head of the pancreas. Note that an endobiliary stent (E) is in situ

Why does this matter?

About half of patients who present with pancreatic cancer are admitted as an emergency either through emergency departments or general practice; this is the highest proportion of GP emergency referrals for any cancer.[11] Only about 11% are referred under the two week wait system for suspected cancer referrals.[11] Patients presenting as emergencies have a lower 12 month survival rate (9%) than those referred under the two week wait rule (19%) or as routine or elective GP referrals (26%).[11] These differences in survival time suggest that the symptoms and signs that currently precipitate a suspected cancer referral are late features.

The age standardised one year survival for pancreatic cancer in England (2005-09) was 17% for men and 19% for women.[12] In the large ESPAC-3 study, resection of the primary tumour followed by adjuvant chemotherapy was associated with a median survival of 43 (95% confidence interval 34 to 56) months, with 29% of patients being alive five years after surgery.[8]

HOW COMMON IS IT?

- In 2012, pancreatic cancer was the 10th most common cancer in the UK and the fifth most common cause of cancer related death[5]
- Incidence is strongly related to age, with a sharp rise after 50-54 years
- In 2011, there were 8773 new cases in the UK: 4328 (49%) in men and 4445 (51%) in women, giving a male:female ratio of almost 1:1[1]
- Incidence and mortality figures are similar, with about 8000 people dying from the disease each year[1]
- Incidence seems to be higher in the Western world, possibly because of the increased prevalence of obesity[6]

Thus, although not all patients with pancreatic cancer are candidates for surgery, evidence suggests that surgery improves survival and earlier diagnosis of non-metastatic tumours may allow more patients to have resection. Earlier diagnosis would also avoid the trauma associated with diagnostic delay.

How is pancreatic cancer diagnosed?

Clinical features

Pancreatic cancer should be considered in any patient with recent onset painless obstructive jaundice. In this setting, management should consist of early referral for further assessment.[13]

Diagnosis is more difficult in patients without jaundice. Here the coexistence of persistent non-specific gastrointestinal symptoms with recent onset or atypical back pain, particularly in the presence of recently diagnosed diabetes or weight loss, should raise an index of suspicion about pancreatic cancer. A large study based on a primary care database developed an algorithm for the diagnosis of pancreatic cancer (table).[14] Independent predictors in both men and women were age, smoking, type 2 diabetes, chronic pancreatitis, abdominal pain, anorexia, and weight loss (table).[14] The 10% of patients with the highest predicted risks made up 62% of all pancreatic cancers diagnosed over the next two years.[14]

A case-control analysis that compared 3635 newly diagnosed patients with age and sex matched controls found that nine features were associated with pancreatic cancer (all $P<0.01$).[15] These were jaundice, abdominal pain, nausea or vomiting, back pain, constipation, diarrhoea, weight loss, malaise, and new onset diabetes.

Investigations

Biochemical liver function tests may help to distinguish between an obstructive and a hepatocellular picture in patients with painless jaundice and guide referral to medical or surgical teams.

Upper abdominal ultrasonography may suggest the diagnosis, but a normal result does not exclude pancreatic cancer.[13] For the diagnosis of pancreatic cancer, ultrasonography has a sensitivity of 90% and specificity of 97%.[16] Ultrasound is operator dependent and false negative results can occur if the pancreas is obscured by gas in the overlying transverse colon.[17]

UK guidelines currently recommend high resolution contrast computed tomography as the diagnostic test of choice.[13] It has a reported sensitivity of 75-100% and a specificity of 70-100% for the diagnosis of pancreatic cancer,[17] although sensitivity for lesions less than 2 cm is only 68-77%.[17] The test also provides information on prognosis by indicating the presence or absence of liver metastasis and invasion of local vascular structures.

How is pancreatic cancer managed?

The modern management of patients with pancreatic cancer requires multidisciplinary care in a high volume specialist centre. In patients with few (or no) comorbidities and a small non-metastatic tumour, current guidelines advocate surgical resection followed by adjuvant chemotherapy.[7]

However, most patients are not candidates for surgery, and supportive care aims to relieve jaundice; establish a tissue diagnosis of cancer; and offer palliative chemotherapy, pancreatic exocrine replacement therapy, adequate analgesia, and palliative care.[7]

Contributors: Both authors reviewed the primary data cited in this article. Both contributed equally to writing the paper. AKS is guarantor.

Competing interests: We have read and understood BMJ policy on declaration of interests and have none to declare.

Provenance and peer review: Commissioned; externally peer reviewed.

Patient consent not required (patient anonymised, hypothetical, or dead).

1 Cancer Research UK. Types of pancreatic cancer. www.cancerresearchuk.org/cancer-help/type/pancreatic-cancer/about/types-of-pancreatic-cancer.
2 Cancer Research UK. Pancreatic cancer symptoms. www.cancerresearchuk.org/cancer-help/type/pancreatic-cancer/about/pancreatic-cancer-symptoms.
3 Watanabe I, Sasaki S, Konishi M, Nakagohri T, Inoue K, Oda T, et al. Onset symptoms and tumor locations as prognostic factors of pancreatic cancer. *Pancreas* 2004;28:160-5.
4 Brennan MF, Moccia RD, Klimstra D. Management of adenocarcinoma of the body and tail of the pancreas. *Ann Surg* 1996;223:506-12.
5 Cancer Research UK. Cancer incidence and mortality in the UK. http://publications.cancerresearchuk.org/downloads/Product/CS_REPORT_TOP10INCMORT.pdf.
6 Simard EP, Ward EM, Siegel R, Jemal A. Cancers with increasing incidence trends in the United States: 1999 through 2008. *CA Cancer J Clin* 2012;62:118-28.
7 National Comprehensive Cancer Network. NCCN clinical practice guidelines in oncology. Pancreatic adenocarcinoma. Version 2. 2014.
8 Neoptolemos JP, Stocken DD, Bassi C, Ghaneh P, Cunningham D, Goldstein D, et al. Adjuvant chemotherapy with fluouracil plus folinic acid versus gemcitabine following pancreatic cancer resection: a randomized controlled trial. *JAMA* 2010;304:1073-81.
9 Sah RP, Nagpal SJS, Mukhopadhyay D, Chari ST. New insights into pancreatic cancer-induced paraneoplastic diabetes. *Nat Rev Gastroenterol Hepatol* 2013;10:423-33.
10 Bond-Smith G, Banga N, Hammond TM, Imber CJ. Pancreatic adenocarcinoma. *BMJ* 2012;344:e2476.
11 National Cancer Intelligence Network. Routes to diagnosis: exploring emergency presentations. 2013. www.ncin.org.uk/publications/data_briefings/routes_to_diagnosis_exploring_emergency_presentations.
12 Cancer Research UK. Pancreatic cancer survival statistics. www.cancerresearchuk.org/cancer-info/cancerstats/types/pancreas/survival/pancreatic-cancer-survival-statistics.
13 Pancreatic section of the British Society of Gastroenterology. Guidelines for the management of patients with pancreatic cancer periampullary and ampullary carcinomas. *Gut* 2005;54 (suppl V):V1-16.
14 Hippisley-Cox J, Coupland C. Identifying patients with suspected pancreatic cancer in primary care: derivation and validation of an algorithm. *Br J Gen Pract* 2012;62:e38-45.
15 Stapley S, Peters TJ, Neal RD, Rose PW, Walter FM, Hamilton W. The risk of pancreatic cancer in symptomatic patients in primary care: a large case-control study using electronic records. *Br J Cancer* 2012;106:1940-4.
16 Karlson B-M, Ekbom A, Lindgren PG, Källskog V, Rastad J. Abdominal US for diagnosis of pancreatic tumor: prospective cohort analysis. *Radiology* 1999;213:107-11.
17 Shrikhande SV, Barreto SG, Goel M, Arya S. Multimodality imaging of pancreatic ductal adenocarcinoma: a review of the literature. 2012;14:658-68.

Multiple myeloma

Danny C Hsu, university lecturer in medical education[1], consultant haematologist[2],
Peter Wilkenfeld, primary care practitioner[3],
Douglas E Joshua, professor of medicine[1], consultant haematologist[2]

[1]University of Sydney, Sydney, NSW 2050, Australia

[2]Institute of Haematology, Royal Prince Alfred Hospital, Sydney, Australia

[3]Bondi Junction, Sydney, NSW 2022, Australia

Correspondence to: D C Hsu danny.hsu@tpg.com.au

Cite this as: *BMJ* 2012;344:d7953

DOI: 10.1136/bmj.d7953

www.bmj.com/content/344/bmj.d7953

A 62 year old man presents to his general practitioner with new onset lower back pain and fatigue for the past few weeks. The patient denies any recent trauma and has otherwise been in good health except for a chest infection treated with oral amoxicillin three months ago. On examination there is midline tenderness over the L5 vertebra with no evidence of neurological signs. The general practitioner requests a full blood count, liver function tests, and a biochemistry panel, which showed mild normocytic normochromic anaemia with rouleaux in the blood film, mild renal impairment, and a raised total protein concentration. Serum electrophoresis confirms the presence of a monoclonal paraprotein. The general practitioner refers the patient to the haematology unit, where myeloma is diagnosed after further investigation and management.

What is multiple myeloma?

Multiple myeloma is a neoplasm of plasma cells characterised by the production of monoclonal immunoglobulin by the malignant cells. This disease predominantly affects older adults, and because of the protean manifestations of the disease patients can initially present to their primary care physicians with vague and confusing symptoms.

Why is multiple myeloma missed?

In a small retrospective UK case review more than half of symptomatic patients who had initially presented to their general practitioners had a delay of more than six months (>12 months in 33% of cases) before specialist referral.[6] A large retrospective review of data from a US cancer registry also confirmed that considerable delays occur in diagnosis, with the median time from onset of symptoms or signs to the diagnosis of myeloma being 99 days.[7] As most patients with myeloma are in their late 60s, they may accept symptoms such as diminished energy, various aches and pains, and slight weight loss as "normal" for their age, especially if symptom onset was gradual.

The protean presentations of myeloma may not initially suggest a haematological diagnosis, especially as non-specific early symptoms such as fatigue, bone pain, and weight loss may overlap with those of more common conditions such as depression, osteoarthritis, and diabetes. In the absence of trauma or neurological symptoms ("red flags"), routine radiography of the back is usually not indicated in the investigation of non-specific back pains. Although no single, specific finding is diagnostic of myeloma, one of the key features of the disease that is often clinically "silent" is the presence of monoclonal paraproteinaemia in blood or urine. The findings of rouleaux (stacks of red cells) in the peripheral blood

KEY POINTS

- The common manifestations of multiple myeloma, such as bone pain, fatigue, and weight loss, may be non-specific and are often initially ignored or missed by patients and medical practitioners
- Early diagnosis of myeloma may prevent debilitating complications such as pathological fractures, irreversible renal impairment, or spinal cord compression
- The finding of rouleaux in the blood film and/or a raised total protein concentration may suggest an underlying paraproteinaemia, especially in a patient with anaemia and bone pain, and would therefore warrant consultation with a haematology specialist

film or a raised erythrocyte sedimentation rate may be the only indications of underlying paraproteinaemia. Therefore, the findings of bone pain associated with renal disease or anaemia with rouleaux may suggest that a haematologist's opinion is necessary.

Why does this matter?

Patients with untreated myeloma can develop debilitating complications such as pathological fractures from lytic lesions, irreversible renal failure requiring long term haemodialysis, or more rarely spinal cord compression from extramedullary plasmacytomas. Delays in diagnosis are associated with a higher rate of complications and reduced disease-free survival.[6] Timely diagnosis of myeloma may prevent the potentially serious complications of the disease.

How is myeloma diagnosed?

Clinical features

The symptoms and signs of myeloma result from malignant plasma cells infiltrating the bones or other organs (such as myelosuppression from marrow infiltration, hepatosplenomegaly), as well as from an increased amount of paraprotein (which causes, for example, hyperviscosity symptoms or paraesthesia from peripheral neuropathy) or light chains in the serum (which result, for example, in renal failure from light chain nephropathy). Patients with early stage disease may remain completely asymptomatic until complications arise. The box lists the most common presenting symptoms or signs, according to a large, single centre retrospective analysis.[8]

Investigations

When myeloma is suspected in a patient, the baseline screening investigations should include:

- A full blood count to detect cytopenias resulting from marrow infiltration
- Inspection of the peripheral blood film to look for rouleaux, which may suggest underlying paraproteinaemia
- Serum biochemistry to detect the presence of renal impairment, hypercalcaemia (from widespread bony destruction, as cytokine expression by myeloma cells results in osteoclastic bone resorption), and raised uric acid (from increased tumour cell turnover)
- Liver function tests to look at the total protein concentration.

At times, the only clue to underlying paraproteinaemia may be an unexpectedly raised total protein concentration, which is brought to the clinician's attention by the clinical chemistry laboratory. A markedly raised erythrocyte sedimentation rate may also suggest the diagnosis of myeloma, with one study showing an average rate of 85 mm/h in newly diagnosed patients.[9] We have to be aware that in patients aged over 50 with a raised erythrocyte sedimentation rate and systemic symptoms, polymyalgia rheumatica is a reasonable differential diagnosis, but treatment with steroids should not be started before considering further investigations to exclude myeloma. The C reactive protein concentration can also be mildly raised in patients with myeloma, but typically it is about 1 mg/dL (9.52 nmol/L) and is not as useful as the erythrocyte sedimentation rate as a screening test. To confirm the presence of monoclonal paraproteins, general practitioners may order serum protein electrophoresis and immunofixation, and serum-free light chains (if available).

As part of the diagnostic investigations after haematology referral, most haematologists would arrange for a bone marrow biopsy to assess the presence of atypical, clonal plasma cells and a 24 hour urine collection for electrophoresis and immunofixation (to detect urinary light chain excretion). Once the diagnosis is confirmed, other tests would include serum immunoglobulin concentrations (to exclude secondary hypogammaglobulinaemia, which may cause recurrent infections) and a radiological skeletal survey (to look for lytic bone lesions).

HOW COMMON IS MULTIPLE MYELOMA?

- In the United Kingdom and the United States myeloma accounts for about 10% of all haematological malignancies[1 2]
- The reported annual incidence of myeloma in the UK and the US is about 3-4 per 100 000[3]
- The incidence of myeloma varies across different ethnic groups; in the US the incidence is twice as high in African Americans as in white people[4] but in ethnic Chinese people in Taiwan it is as low as 0.75 per 100 000[5]

MOST COMMON PRESENTING SYMPTOMS OR SIGNS[8]

- Normochromic, normocytic anaemia—about 70% of patients
- Bone pain—about 60%
- Renal impairment—about 50%
- Fatigue—about 30%
- Weight loss—about 25%
- Hypercalcaemia—about 15%
- Hyperviscosity symptoms*—<7%
- Paraesthesia—5%
- Spinal cord compression—5%
- Hepatomegaly—4%
- Splenomegaly—1%
- Lymphadenopathy—1%
- Fever <1%

**Such as headache, visual disturbance, cognitive impairment*

In 97% of patients with myeloma, the combination of serum and urine electrophoresis and immunofixation can detect a monoclonal paraprotein (M protein). Serum or urine electrophoresis is used to quantitate the amount of detectable paraprotein, whereas immunofixation is used to confirm the monoclonal nature of the protein as well as characterise the specific immunoglobulin subclass. It is important to note that other plasma cell disorders (such as plasmacytomas) and lymphoproliferative disorders (such as chronic lymphocytic leukaemia and non-Hodgkin's lymphoma) can also be associated with an M protein.

To diagnose symptomatic myeloma, three diagnostic criteria must be fulfilled[10]:

1. The presence of an M protein in serum or urine (no specific cut-off as 40% of symptomatic patients with myeloma will have a level <30 g/L)
2. The presence of >10% clonal plasma cells in the bone marrow aspirate
3. Evidence of end organ damage (the so called CRAB features of hyper**C**alcaemia from bone destruction, **R**enal impairment, **A**naemia, and lytic **B**one lesions on imaging).

Patients who meet criteria 1 and 2 without evidence of the CRAB features are said to have smouldering myeloma. An asymptomatic patient (without CRAB features) whose bone marrow biopsy shows <10% plasma cells or whose serum or urinary M protein concentrations are <30 g/L has monoclonal gammopathy of undetermined significance. This condition is much more common than myeloma, with an estimated prevalence of 3% in the general population aged over 50 years.[11] This premalignant condition confers a risk of progression into myeloma (or into related lymphoproliferative disorders) of 1% a year.

How is myeloma managed?

Refer patients with suspected myeloma to a specialist haematology unit for further investigation and management. Conventionally, after confirmation of the diagnosis with tests including a diagnostic bone marrow biopsy and skeletal survey, patients with evidence of end organ damage need treatment. Patients with smouldering myeloma are generally monitored closely as historically there has been no evidence that early treatment of these patients confers a superior long term outcome. However, with the development of new therapeutic agents with more favourable toxicity profiles, there are now phase III trials challenging this dogma and looking at the outcomes of early treatment of patients with monoclonal gammopathy of undetermined significance or smouldering myeloma.

Patients with myeloma are broadly divided into two main groups: those who are or are not eligible for an autologous stem cell transplant. This division is important as cytotoxic agents form the backbone of modern treatment for myeloma, and in patients eligible for transplantation the excessive use of alkylating agents may jeopardise a successful stem cell collection. Patients often receive repeated cycles of induction chemotherapy—usually in combination with thalidomide, lenalidomide, or bortezomib—before stem cell mobilisation and autologous transplantation.

Patients who are not eligible for transplantation are typically treated with combination chemotherapy until resolution of end organ damage and absence of detectable paraprotein. All patients with myeloma require bisphosphonates, which reduce pathological fractures and skeletal related events in myeloma.[12] A recent randomised controlled trial suggests that zoledronic acid may be the bisphosphonate of choice.[13] Adjuvant treatments in the form of localised radiotherapy may also be used for patients with symptomatic lytic lesions. Patients with recurrent infections resulting from secondary hypogammaglobulinaemia may benefit from regular intravenous immunoglobulin replacement.

Contributors: DEJ proposed the overall concept of the article and is the guarantor. DCH did the literature search. All authors contributed to writing the article.

Competing interests: All authors have completed the ICMJE uniform disclosure form at www.icmje.org/coi_disclosure.pdf (available on request from the corresponding author) and declare: no support from any organisation for the submitted work; no financial relationships with any organisations that might have an interest in the submitted work in the previous three years; no other relationships or activities that could appear to have influenced the submitted work.

Provenance and peer review: Commissioned; externally peer reviewed.

Patient consent not required (patient anonymised, dead, or hypothetical).

1 Office for National Statistics. Cancer Statistics registrations: registrations of cancer diagnosed in 2008, England. (Series MB1 no 39.) 2010. National Statistics. www.ons.gov.uk/ons/rel/vsob1/cancer-statistics-registrations--england--series-mb1-/no--39--2008/index.html.
2 Jemal A, Siegel R, Ward E, Hao Y, Xu J, Thun MJ. Cancer statistics, 2009. *CA Cancer J Clin* 2009;59:225-49.
3 Phekoo KJ, Schey SA, Richards MA, Bevan DH, Bell S, Gillett D, et al. A population study to define the incidence and survival of multiple myeloma in a National Health Service region in UK. *Br J Haematol* 2004;127:299-304.
4 Waxman AJ, Mink PJ, Devesa SS, Anderson WF, Weiss BM, Kristinsson SY, et al. Racial disparities in incidence and outcome in multiple myeloma: a population-based study. *Blood* 2010;116:5501-6.
5 Huang SY, Yao M, Tang JL, Lee WC, Tsay W, Cheng AL, et al. Epidemiology of multiple myeloma in Taiwan: increasing incidence for the past 25 years and higher prevalence of extramedullary myeloma in patients younger than 55 years. *Cancer* 2007;110:896-905.
6 Kariyawasan CC, Hughes DA, Jayatillake MM, Mehta AB. Multiple myeloma: causes and consequences of delay in diagnosis. *QJM* 2007;100:635-40.
7 Friese CR, Abel GA, Magazu LS, Neville BA, Richardson LS, Earle CC. Diagnostic delay and complications for older adults with multiple myeloma. *Leuk Lymphoma* 2009;50:392-400.
8 Kyle RA, Gertz MA, Witzig TE, Lust JA, Lacy MQ, Dispenzieri A, et al. Review of 1027 patients with newly diagnosed multiple myeloma. Mayo Clin Proc 2003;78:21-33.
9 Alexandrakis MG, Passam FH, Ganotakis ES, Sfiridaki K, Xilouri I, Perisinakis K, et al. The clinical and prognostic significance of erythrocyte sedimentation rate (ESR), serum interleukin-6 (IL-6) and acute phase protein levels in multiple myeloma. *Clin Lab Haem* 2003;25:41-6.

10 International Myeloma Working Group. Criteria for the classification of monoclonal gammopathies, multiple myeloma and related disorders: a report of the International Myeloma Working Group. *Br J Haematol* 2003;121:749-57.
11 Kyle RA, Rajkumar SV. Monoclonal gammopathy of undetermined significance and smouldering multiple myeloma: emphasis on risk factors for progression. *Br J Haematol* 2007;139:730-43.
12 Mhaskar R, Redzepovic J, Wheatley K, Clark OA, Miladinovic B, Glasmacher A, et al. Bisphosphonates in multiple myeloma. *Cochrane Database Syst Rev* 2010;3:CD003188.
13 Morgan GJ, Davies FE, Gregory WM, Cocks K, Bell SE, Szubert AJ, et al. First-line treatment with zoledronic acid as compared with clodronic acid in multiple myeloma (MRC Myeloma IX): a randomised controlled trial. *Lancet* 2010;376:1989-99.

Bladder cancer in women

Brian D Nicholson, academic clinical fellow in primary care[1],
John S McGrath, consultant urological surgeon[2],
honorary senior lecturer[3],
Willie Hamilton, professor of primary care diagnostics[3]

[1]Department of Primary Health Care Services, Oxford University, Oxford OX2 6GG, UK

[2]Royal Devon and Exeter NHS Foundation Trust, Exeter, UK

[3]University of Exeter Medical School, Exeter EX2 4SG, UK

Correspondence to: B D Nicholson brian.nicholson@phc.ox.ac.uk

Cite this as: *BMJ* 2014;348:g2171

<DOI> 10.1136/bmj.g2171

www.bmj.com/content/348/bmj.g2171

A 76 year old woman reports recurrent urinary frequency, dysuria, and malodorous urine. No bacterial growth has been identified on two midstream urine samples, though empirical treatment with antibiotics has improved her symptoms. After three months, an episode of visible haematuria prompts referral and a transitional cell carcinoma of the bladder is diagnosed.

What are the types of bladder cancer?

In developed countries 90% of bladder cancers are transitional cell carcinomas; squamous cell carcinomas (SCC) make up most of the remainder.[1 2] In endemic areas, squamous cell carcinoma related to schistosomiasis accounts for 70% of cases.[1] Around 20% are muscle invasive at diagnosis and are associated with a significantly poorer prognosis.[3] The major risk factor is smoking, though chronic infection, radiotherapy, and (before regulation) industrial dyes have been implicated.[2 4]

Why is it missed?

Although bladder cancer is more common in men, women experience more delays: the English National Audit of Cancer Diagnosis in Primary Care (2009-10) estimated that annually 435 more women than men with bladder cancer experience a delay in diagnosis, but there are few data from UK primary care to explain this.[6] With no effective screening tool for bladder cancer, it is usually diagnosed symptomatically, with haematuria being the most common presenting symptom for both sexes in primary care (likelihood ratio 59, 95% confidence interval 51 to 57).[3 7] The likelihood ratio summarises how many times more (or less) likely patients with bladder cancer are to have a particular feature than patients without bladder cancer. A ratio over 10 (or under 0.1) is considered to provide strong evidence to rule in (or rule out) bladder cancer.

A study of outpatient haematuria claims for 7649 patients aged >65 in the United States (female:male 1:2.43) also described a delay in diagnosis after presentation in women. The mean time to diagnosis was 85.5 days in women (95% confidence interval 81.3 to 89.4) compared with 73.6 days (71.2 to 76.1) in men (P<0.001). This difference persisted over time; women were 26% more likely to experience delay at three months after the initial claim, 16% at six months, and 23% at nine months.[8] During investigations, women undergo more urinalyses (1.39 *v* 1.19, P<0.001) and urine cultures (0.83 *v* 0.53, P<0.001) and receive more diagnoses of urinary tract infections (odds ratio 2.32, 95% confidence interval 2.07 to 2.59;

KEY POINTS

- Women with bladder cancer are more likely to present with muscle invasive disease, partly associated with delays in diagnosis in primary care
- Haematuria is the most highly predictive symptom of bladder cancer, and appropriate investigation and referral should not be delayed
- If women are treated for presumed urinary tract infection, active follow-up should ensure that symptoms have settled with treatment with antibiotics
- Symptomatic women aged over 50 without confirmation of infection on urinalysis or microscopy and culture should be referred for further assessment to identify a definitive cause

P<0.001) and more antibiotics (40.1% v 35.4%, P<0.001), yet are less likely to undergo bladder imaging (odds ratio 0.80, 0.71 to 0.89; P<0.001).[8]

Bladder cancer is also associated with voiding disorders and abdominal pain, but European data from primary care and gynaecology report that women with these complaints are more likely to be treated empirically, with treatments given without further evaluation in 47% of women compared with 19% of men in the year before diagnosis (P<0.05).[9]

Although these data are not wholly derived from primary care, it is implicit that prolonged investigation and treatment for urinary tract infections over repeated consultations (without confirmation of symptom resolution) is more of a problem in women.

Why does this matter?

Although there are recognised sex differences in tumour biology, bladder anatomy, and environmental and hormonal exposures that contribute to differential outcomes, there is some evidence of a correlation between delay in primary care and worsening prognosis.[10 11 12]

Prospective data from the UK for 1537 cases of bladder cancer (1340 detailing stage, and 633 both stage and cause of death) showed an association between longer delay between start of symptoms and GP referral and a 5% increased incidence of muscle invasive bladder cancer (pT2-4) (P=0.04).[12] Five year survival was significantly worse for women presenting with muscle invasive disease (P<0.001).[12] While the report did not distinguish between patient delay and GP delay, longer delay before referral (>14 v <14 days) resulted in an increased risk of death (hazard ratio 1.19, 95% confidence interval 1.01 to 1.42; P=0.04) and 5% poorer five year survival (P=0.02).[12] Patients with delay in their referral pathway seem to have more advanced disease, with poorer outcomes; arguably, they warrant the most expedient intervention compared with other groups.

How is it diagnosed?

Clinical features

The National Institute for Health and Care Excellence (NICE) recommends urgent urology referral for adults with visible haematuria in the absence of urinary tract infection or in the presence of recurrent or persistent urinary tract infection in those aged >40; for unexplained microscopic haematuria in those aged >50; and for an abdominal mass arising from the bladder; and a non-urgent referral in those aged <50 with unexplained microscopic haematuria without raised creatinine concentration or proteinuria.[13]

Most studies in primary care have examined haematuria alone, though two—which both used pre-existing medical records—reported a broad range of symptoms associated with bladder cancer per se[3] and with urinary tract cancer collectively.[14] Most patients presented with painless haematuria, voiding symptoms, or a combination of the two.

Haematuria

The case-control study using electronic medical records from UK primary care showed that painless macroscopic haematuria is the strongest predictor of bladder cancer in primary care (odds ratio 34, 95% confidence interval 29 to 41), with a positive predictive value in patients aged over 60 of 3.9% (3.5% to 4.6%).[3] The national audit showed that two thirds of patients had haematuria recorded as their primary symptom in primary care[6]; though the prospective secondary care study showed that 90% of referred patients had haematuria (the severity of which did not correlate with disease severity); 25% of those referred will have transitional cell carcinoma of the bladder.[6 12]

Less specific symptoms

The case-control study also showed that the commonly encountered symptoms of dysuria (odds ratio 4.1, 95% confidence interval 3.4 to 5.0), abdominal pain (2.0, 1.6 to 2.4), and constipation (1.5, 1.2 to 1.9), and a diagnosis of urinary tract infection (2.2, 2.0 to 2.5) are associated with bladder cancer but with much lower predictive values.[3] Patients with more

HOW COMMON IS BLADDER CANCER IN WOMEN?

- Bladder cancer is the seventh most common cancer in the United Kingdom and the 11th most common in women[5]
- In 2010 there were 10324 new diagnoses of bladder cancer in the UK, with a female to male ratio of 2:5, accounting for 4900 deaths[5]
- An average general practice expects to see one new diagnosis of female bladder cancer every 3.5 years
- The average age at diagnosis is 71[5]

advanced disease might present with pelvic pain or urinary obstruction. In these patients, a mass might be palpable. Importantly, re-attendance with persistent symptoms is associated with an increased risk of cancer.

Investigations

Non-specific

Urinalysis is accurate in detecting haematuria, proteinuria, nitrites, or leucocyte esterase, with subsequent microscopy and culture to confirm infection. Although three blood tests with abnormal results—raised white cell count, raised inflammatory markers, and raised creatinine—are associated with bladder cancer, these tests alone cannot be used to rule out the condition.[3] The main role of urine cytology is in follow-up of patients with carcinoma in situ, rather than in the diagnosis of cancer. No primary care studies have reported its performance characteristics in diagnosis, but sensitivity is only 38% in secondary care and probably lower in primary care.[15]

Definitive

Flexible cystoscopy is the mainstay of investigation and is performed on a day case basis. It allows direct visualisation and biopsy of bladder abnormalities, but not treatment. Ultrasongraphy of the renal tract is often added as the symptoms of bladder and renal cancer overlap.[6] For patients with bladder cancer, staging might require computerised tomography and isotope bone scanning; positron emission tomography is increasingly used in specialist centres.

How is it managed?

Initial treatment depends on staging; less advanced disease is resected transurethrally (TURBT). Patients with low risk disease are offered cystoscopic surveillance, while recurrent low risk disease or intermediate/high risk disease can require intravesical chemotherapy or immunotherapy (with BCG). More advanced disease can require cystectomy or radical radiotherapy, with or without neo-adjuvant chemotherapy.[2]

Contributors: BDN performed the initial searches and drafted the first version of the article. All authors revised the article, adding additional references. WH is guarantor.

Competing interests: We have read and understood the BMJ policy on declaration of interests and declare the following interests: WH has had many research grants relating to cancer diagnostics from non-commercial sources, including an NIHR programme grant which incorporates a bladder cancer study. He is the clinical lead for the current revision of the NICE 2005 guidance (CG 27) on the topic of selection of patients for cancer investigation. His contribution to this article is in a personal capacity and is not to be interpreted as representing the view of the Guideline Development Group or NICE. He has received travel support to give lectures and attend conferences, plus occasional speaker's fees, from conference organisers in the charitable and educational sector, though none from commercial sources. BDN is funded by the National Institute for Health Research (NIHR) School for Primary Care Research (SPCR). The views expressed are those of the author(s) and not necessarily those of the NHS, the NIHR, or the Department of Health.

Provenance and peer review: Not commissioned; externally peer reviewed.

Patient consent: Not required (hypothetical).

1 Kaufman DS, Shipley WU, Feldman AS. Bladder cancer. *Lancet* 2009;374:239-49.

2 Lunt CR, Maddineni SB, Brough R. Bladder cancer. *Br J Med Surg Urol* 2012;5:95-103.

3 Shephard EA, Stapley S, Neal RD, Rose P, Walter FM, Hamilton WT. Clinical features of bladder cancer in primary care. *Br J Gen Pract* 2012;62:e598-604.

4 Jemal A, Bray F, Center MM, Ferlay J, Ward E, Forman D. Global cancer statistics. *CA Cancer J Clin* 2011;61:69-90.

5 Bladder cancer. Cancer Research UK, 2013. www.cancerresearchuk.org/cancer-help/type/bladder-cancer/

6 Lyratzopoulos G, Abel GA, McPhail S, Neal RD, Rubin GP. Gender inequalities in the promptness of diagnosis of bladder and renal cancer after symptomatic presentation: evidence from secondary analysis of an English primary care audit survey. *BMJ Open* 2013;3:e002861.

7 Allaby M. Screening for bladder cancer using the urinalysis/dipstick method: a report for the national screening committee. NHS, 2010. www.screening.nhs.uk/policydb_download.php?doc=62

8 Cohn JA, Vekhter B, Lyttle C, Steinberg GD, Large MC. Sex disparities in diagnosis of bladder cancer after initial presentation with hematuria. *Cancer* 2013;120:555-61.

9 Henning A, Wehrberger M, Madersbacher S, Pycha A, Martini T, Comploj E, et al. Do differences in clinical symptoms and referral patterns contribute to the gender gap in bladder cancer? *BJU Int* 2013;112:68-73.

10 Fajkovic H, Halpern JA, Cha EK, Bahadori A, Chromecki TF, Karakiewicz PI, et al. Impact of gender on bladder cancer incidence, staging, and prognosis. *World J Urol* 2011;29:457-63.

11 Shariat SF, Sfakianos JP, Droller MJ, Karakiewicz PI, Meryn S, Bochner BH. The effect of age and gender on bladder cancer: a critical review of the literature. *BJU Int* 2010;105:300-8.

12 Wallace DM, Bryan RT, Dunn JA, Begum G, Bathers S, on behalf of the West Midlands Urological Research Group. Delay and survival in bladder cancer. *BJU Int* 2002;89:868-78.

13 NICE. Referral for suspected cancer (CG27). National Institute for Health and Care Excellence, 2005.

14 Hippisley-Cox J, Coupland C. Identifying patients with suspected renal tract cancer in primary care: derivation and validation of an algorithm. *Br J Gen Pract* 2012;62:e251-60.

15 Planz B, Jochims E, Deix T, Caspers HP, Jakse G, Boecking A. The role of urinary cytology for detection of bladder cancer. *Eur J Surg Oncol* 2005;31:304-8.

Metastatic spinal cord compression

Nasir A Quraishi, consultant spine surgeon[1],
Claire Esler, consultant oncologist[2]

[1]Centre for Spine Studies and Surgery, Queen's Medical Centre, Nottingham NG7 2UH, UK

[2]Department of Oncology, Leicester Royal Infirmary, Leicester, UK

Correspondence to: N A Quraishi nasquraishi@hotmail.com

Cite this as: *BMJ* 2011;342:d2402

DOI: 10.1136/bmj.d2402

www.bmj.com/content/342/bmj.d2402

Metastatic spinal cord compression is defined radiographically as an epidural metastatic lesion causing true displacement of the spinal cord from its normal position in the spinal canal.[1] It is an important source of morbidity (including paralysis and bowel and bladder disorders) in patients with systemic cancer.

Why is metastatic spinal cord compression missed?

Low back pain is one of the most common complaints in primary care, with most cases being benign, self limiting, and not needing a specific diagnosis. The challenge in primary care is therefore to identify those cases where low back pain is caused by a serious spinal disease, such as malignancy. Low back pain may be the first presentation of malignancy, and about 23% of patients with spinal metastases are thought to have had no previous diagnosis of cancer.[4]

In a prospective observational study of 319 patients with metastatic cord compression, a median of two months passed from the onset of pain as reported to their primary care providers until the diagnosis of metastatic cord compression.[5] Therefore, new onset back or neck pain in a patient with known cancer must be considered to be spinal metastatic disease until proved otherwise.

Why does it matter?

Although the rate of clinical progression is variable, patients with motor dysfunction inevitably progress to complete paralysis in the absence of intervention.[6] Almost half of patients cannot walk by the time of diagnosis.[7] However, neurological status at the time of diagnosis, particularly motor function, has been shown to correlate with prognosis from metastatic cord compression,[8] thus reinforcing the concept that diagnosis before the development of a neurological deficit is of paramount importance. Furthermore, treatment before paralysis is clinically and cost effective.[9]

How is it diagnosed?

Clinical features

All segments of the spine can be affected by metastatic cord compression, but the thoracic spine is the most commonly affected site (about 70% of cases), followed by the lumbar spine (20%), cervical spine, and sacrum.[6] As thoracic pain is less common in the general population than pain originating from the mobile cervical and lumbar regions, pain in the thorax should increase suspicion of the likelihood of cancer.[10]

KEY POINTS

- New onset back or neck pain in a patient with known cancer must be considered to be spinal metastatic disease until proved otherwise
- If metastatic cord compression is suspected, urgent specialist referral is critical as early diagnosis and treatment improves quality of life and functional outcome, such as the prevention of paraplegia
- Magnetic resonance imaging is the optimal imaging modality for assessing spinal metastatic disease
- Initial treatment includes corticosteroid use, with urgent definitive treatment comprising surgery or radiotherapy

Indeed pain is the most common presenting symptom of spinal metastases, occurring in 83-95% of cases.[7] Three classic pain syndromes affect patients with spinal metastases: *(a)* local pain, with pain at rest (resulting from periosteal stretching from tumour growth and/or local inflammatory processes); *(b)* mechanical pain, with pain on movement and improved by rest (owing to instability); and *(c)* radicular pain (owing to irritation of a nerve root).[7] Patients will often present with a combination of these, and they may have both myelopathic (with long tract signs such as upper motor neurone signs) and radicular abnormalities. They may have lower extremity weakness and hyper-reflexia below the level of compression (hyporeflexia if the cauda equina is compressed).

Sensory changes such as paraesthesia or anaesthesia typically occur in correlation with motor weakness. Patients may therefore complain of sensory abnormalities in the same dermatomal distribution as their motor dysfunction, and patients with myelopathy may describe a sensory change across the chest or abdomen. Patients may also have some degree of dysfunction of the bladder, bowel, and sexual organs as a result of metastatic cord compression. Of these autonomic findings (present in 40-64% of patients with metastatic cord compression),[11] bladder dysfunction is the most common and often correlates with the degree of motor dysfunction.[10] Sensory and autonomic symptoms and signs present late in these patients, and clinicians must therefore have a low suspicion threshold if patients with known malignancy have back pain. In the United Kingdom the guidelines from the National Institute for Health and Clinical Excellence (NICE) recommend education of patients at risk of developing metastatic spinal cord compression so that they know what symptoms to look out for.[12]

Investigations

A general practitioner who suspects a patient of having metastatic spinal cord compression must immediately contact a specialist spine or oncology team for consideration of urgent imaging and further management. The NICE guidelines recommend that centres treating patients with this condition have a coordinator who advises clinicians, coordinates care, and organises urgent magnetic resonance imaging (fig 1 and fig 2).[12] Such imaging remains the optimal imaging modality for assessing spinal metastatic disease (sensitivity 44-100%, specificity 90-93%).[13 14]

How is it managed?

Metastatic spinal cord compression is an oncological emergency and, once it has been radiologically confirmed, definitive treatment should ideally start within 24 hours of diagnosis. Patients may have considerable pain and should receive analgesia in accordance with the World Health Organization's "pain ladder" (http://who.int/cancer/palliative/painladder/en/). NICE guidelines showed, on the basis of a systematic review of low quality randomised controlled trials and observational studies, that corticosteroids (dexamethasone 16 mg daily with gastric protection) may result in rapid improvement of neurological function.[12 15 16]

Primary treatment depends on a patient's performance status, prognosis, preference, and tumour histological type. In very frail, terminally ill patients, active treatment may not be appropriate. Most patients are not suitable for surgery and should receive urgent external beam radiotherapy, although systematic reviews give no clear consensus on the best radiotherapy dose and fractionation.[17] Patients with paraplegia are unlikely to regain any function, and treatment is mainly intended to help with pain.

On the basis of a systematic review from the NICE guidelines of moderate to low quality evidence from retrospective studies,[18 19 20 21] one prospective non-comparative study,[22] one randomised controlled study,[23] and an indirect comparative meta-analysis,[24] surgery may provide better patient outcomes (including pain relief, a better chance of neurological recovery, and maintenance of ambulation) than radiotherapy in carefully selected patients.[12] NICE therefore recommends surgery (decompression and stabilisation) plus radiotherapy for

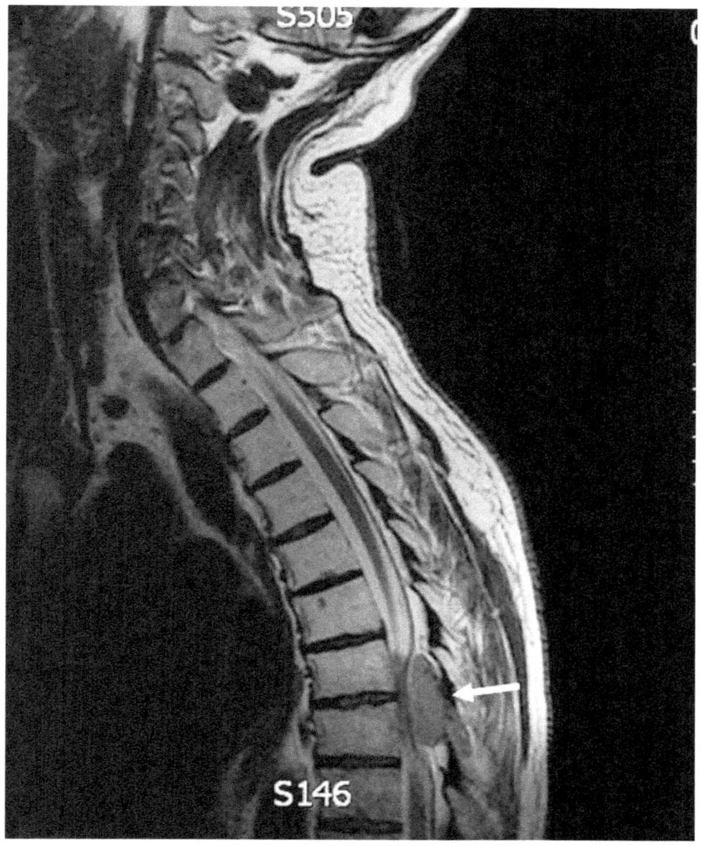

Fig 1 T2 weighted sagittal magnetic resonance scan showing metastatic spinal cord compression by a mass at T7-T8 (arrow)

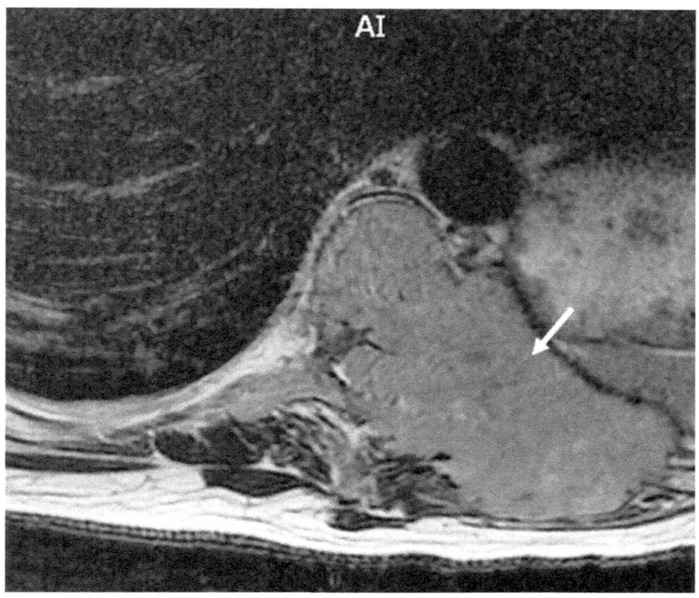

Fig 2 Axial magnetic resonance scan at the T7-T8 level showing extensive tumour infiltration (arrow) with almost complete compression of the spinal cord

patients who are fit enough for surgery, have a prognosis of at least three months, and have:

- Spinal cord compression and have not had paraplegia for more than 48 hours, or
- An unstable spine, or
- Deteriorating neurological function, or
- Pain despite previous radiotherapy.[12]

CASE SCENARIO

A 58 year old woman presents to her general practitioner with a two month history of middle to low back pain. She has a history of breast carcinoma, diagnosed eight years previously and which was treated with a mastectomy and chemotherapy. She also describes pins and needles in both legs for the past three days. On examination, she has tenderness over the area of the T11 and T12 vertebrae and reduced power distally (T4 and T5) but intact bowel and bladder function. She is referred urgently to the metastatic cord compression coordinator, who organises magnetic resonance imaging, which shows cord compression by a mass at the T11 and T12 levels, thought to be caused by metastases.

HOW COMMON IS METASTATIC SPINAL CORD COMPRESSION?

- Skeletal system metastases are the third most common metastases, after those of the pulmonary and hepatic systems[2]
- Within the skeletal system, the spinal column is the most common site of metastases[2]
- Metastatic cord compression is estimated to occur in 5-10% of patients with cancer (most commonly those with breast, prostate, and lung cancers) and in about 40% of patients who have pre-existing, non-spinal bone metastases[3]
- Symptomatic metastatic spinal disease is expected to become more prevalent as survival rates for many common cancers improve

Chemotherapy may occasionally be used as a primary treatment for metastatic cord compression that results from chemosensitive disease such as small cell lung cancer and lymphomas. Whatever treatment a patient receives, ongoing multidisciplinary care is crucial, attending to the patient's medical, social, and psychological needs. Although rehabilitation is important for some patients, palliative care is crucial, as only about a fifth of patients with metastatic cord compression will survive for more than one year.[12]

Contributors: NAQ drafted the original paper and revised the article and added images. CE helped with editing and subsequent drafts.

Competing interests: Both authors have completed the Unified Competing Interest form at www.icmje.org/coi_disclosure.pdf and declare no support from any organisation for the submitted work; no relationships with any companies that might have an interest in the submitted work in the previous 3 years; and no non-financial interests that may be relevant to the submitted work.

Provenance and peer review: Not commissioned; externally peer reviewed.

Patient consent not required (patient anonymised, dead, or hypothetical).

1 Loblaw DA, Laperriere NJ, Mackillop WJ. A population based study of malignant spinal cord compression in Ontario. *Clin Oncol* 2003;14:472-80.
2 Aaron AD.The management of cancer metastatic to bone. *JAMA* 1994;272:1206-9.
3 Schaberg J, Gainor BJ. A profile of metastatic carcinoma of the spine. *Spine* 1985;10:19-20.
4 Levack P, Graham J, Collie D, Grant R, Kidd J, Kunkler I, et al. Don't wait for a sensory level—listen to the symptoms: a prospective audit of the delays in diagnosis of malignant cord compression. *Clin Oncol (R Coll Radiol)* 2002;14:472-80.
5 Levack P, Collie D, Gibson A, Graham J, Grant R, Hurman D, et al. A prospective audit of the diagnosis, management and outcome of malignant cord compression. (Report No CRAG 97/08.) 2001. www.crag.scot.nhs.uk/committees/ceps/reports/F%20Report%20copy%206-2-02.PDF.
6 Helweg-Larsen S, Sorensen PS. Symptoms and signs in metastatic spinal cord compression: a study from first symptom until diagnosis in 153 patients. *Eur J Cancer* 1994;30A:396-8.
7 Quraishi NA, Gokaslan ZL, Boriani S. Review article: the surgical management of metastatic epidural compression of the spinal cord. *J Bone Joint Surg (Br)* 2010;92:1054-60.
8 Schiff D. Spinal cord compression. *Neurological Clinics* 2003;21(1):67-86.
9 White BD, Stirling AJ, Paterson E, Asquith-Coe K, Melder A. Diagnosis and management of patients at risk of or with metastatic spinal cord compression: summary of NICE guidance. *BMJ* 2008;337:a2538.
10 Sciubba DM, Gokaslan ZL. Diagnosis and management of metastatic spine disease. *Surg Oncol* 2006;15:141-51.
11 Young K, Tibbs PA, Patchell RA. Clinical approach to metastatic epidural spinal cord compression. *Hematol Oncol Clin N Am* 2006;20:1297-305.

12 National Institute for Health and Clinical Excellence. Metastatic spinal cord compression: diagnosis and management of patients at risk of or with metastatic spinal cord compression. (Clinical guideline 75.) 2008. www.nice.org.uk/CG75

13 Baur A, Stäbler A, Arbogast S, Duerr HR, Bartl R, Reiser M.Acute osteoporotic and neoplastic vertebral compression fractures: fluid sign at MR imaging. *Radiology* 2002;225:730-5.

14 Jung HS, Jee WH, McCauley TR, Ha KY, Choi KH. Discrimination of metastatic from acute osteoporotic compression fractures with MR imaging. *Radiographics* 2003;23:179-87.

15 Sorensen S, Helweg-Larsen S, Mouridsen H, Hansen HH. Effect of high-dose dexamethasone in carcinomatous metastatic spinal cord compression treated with radiotherapy: a randomised trial. *Eur J Cancer* 1994;30A:22-7.

16 Graham PH, Capp A, Delaney G, Goozee G, Hickey B, Turner S, et al. A pilot randomised comparison of dexamethasone 96 mg vs 16 mg per day for malignant spinal-cord compression treated by radiotherapy: TROG 01.05 Superdex study. *Clin Oncol* 2006;18:70-6.

17 Prewett S, Venkitaraman R. Metastatic spinal cord compression: review of the evidence for a radiotherapy dose fractionation schedule. *Clin Oncol* 2010;22:222-30.

18 Chen YJ, Chang GC, Chen HT, Yang TY, Kuo BI, Hsu HC, et al. Surgical results of metastatic spinal cord compression secondary to non-small cell lung cancer. *Spine* 2007;32:E413-8.

19 Senel A, Kaya AH, Kuroglu E, Celik F. Circumferential stabilisation with ghost screwing after posterior resection of spinal metastases via transpedicular route. *Neurosurg Rev* 2007;30:131-7.

20 Shehadi JA, Sciubba DM, Suk I, Suki D, Maldaun MVC, McCutcheon IE, et al. Surgical treatment strategies and outcome in patients with breast cancer metastatic to the spine: a review of 87 patients. *Eur Spine J* 2007;16:1179-92.

21 Witham TF, Khavkin YA, Gallia GL, Wolinsky JP, Gokaslan ZL. Surgery insight: current management of epidural spinal cord compression from metastatic spine disease. *Nat Clin Pract Neurol* 2006;2(2):87-94.

22 Mannion RJ, Wilby M, Godward S, Lyratzopoulos G, Laing RJC. The surgical management of metastatic spinal disease: prospective assessment and long-term follow-up. *Br J Neurosurg* 2007;21:593-8.

23 Patchell RA, Tibbs PA, Regine WF, Payne R, Saris S, Kryscio RJ, et al. Direct decompressive surgical resection in the treatment of spinal cord compression caused by metastatic cancer: a randomized trial. *Lancet* 2005;6:643-8.

24 Klimo P Jr, Kestle JR, Schmidt MH. Treatment of metastatic spinal epidural disease: a review of the literature. *Neurosurgical Focus* 2003;15: E1.

Carcinoid syndrome

R Srirajaskanthan, specialist registrar[1],
D Shanmugabavan, general practitioner[2],
J K Ramage, consultant gastroenterologist[1]

[1]Institute of Liver Studies, King's College Hospital, London SE5 9RS

[2]Bexley Care Trust, Bexley Heath DA7 6HZ

Correspondence to: R Srirajaskanthan r.srirajaskanthan@nhs.net

Cite this as: *BMJ* 2010;341:c3941

DOI: 10.1136/bmj.c3941

www.bmj.com/content/341/bmj.c3941

Carcinoid syndrome consists of symptoms of facial flushing, diarrhoea, and episodic abdominal pain.[1] It is caused by kinins and serotonin secreted from neuroendocrine tumours that arise from neuroendocrine cells found in almost all organs of the body, most commonly the gastrointestinal tract. Only 30-40% of neuroendocrine tumours cause clinical syndromes; ileal neuroendocrine tumours most commonly cause carcinoid syndrome. Over 95% of patients with carcinoid syndrome have metastatic disease. Hormones secreted by the primary tumour are metabolised by the liver and so do not cause symptoms, but symptoms may develop with liver metastases, as these release hormones that bypass the enterohepatic circulation and enter the systemic circulation.

Why is it missed?

The average time from presentation to diagnosis is four to seven years.[5 6] Symptoms are similar to those in more common conditions, primarily irritable bowel syndrome. In women over 40, the facial flushing is sometimes thought to be a sign of the menopause. Patients are often sent for investigation of diarrhoea, including gastroscopy and colonoscopy, which rarely identifies a primary neuroendocrine tumour because the tumours are small and usually located in the ileum. Unlike patients with other gastrointestinal cancers that may progress rapidly, patients with neuroendocrine tumours may seem well. Consequently clinicians often do not refer these patients for computed tomography or ultrasound, which delays diagnosis. The low incidence of neuroendocrine tumours may also contribute to lower awareness of the condition among primary and secondary care doctors.

Why does it matter?

More than 95% of patients with carcinoid syndrome will have liver metastases with a primary tumour in the small bowel. Surgical resection of the primary tumour and the liver metastases may be possible in the early stages,[7] but late diagnosis may mean that the disease has progressed further, making the tumours inoperable. Surgical resection offers a survival benefit (43 (SD 26.1) months) compared to palliative treatments such as hepatic chemoembolisation (24 (15.8) months).[8] Earlier diagnosis will enable treatment of carcinoid syndrome with somatostatin analogues, but these can be debilitating for some patients.

KEY POINTS

- Carcinoid syndrome results from kinins and serotonin released from neuroendocrine tumours, most commonly those in the gastrointestinal tract. Its most common symptoms are facial flushing, diarrhoea, and cramping abdominal pain
- Delayed diagnosis may lead to progression of disease and consequently shorter survival from time of diagnosis
- Urinary 5-HIAA and abdominal ultrasound are initial investigations in primary care; foods containing tyramine should be excluded at least 24 hours before urine collection
- Carcinoid syndrome can be treated with somatostatin analogues or interferon alfa, or both. Surgery is the only option with curative potential for neuroendocrine tumours

CASE SCENARIO

A 40 year old man presented with a three year history of diarrhoea and episodic abdominal pain with no clear precipitating factors. After coeliac disease was excluded a provisional diagnosis of irritable bowel syndrome was made and various treatments were tried, without benefit. Over the past year his wife and children had noticed intermittent facial flushing. Ultrasound of the abdomen, performed by his general practitioner for his persistent abdominal cramping, identified liver lesions. On referral to a gastroenterologist, 5-hydroxyindoleacetic acid (5HIAA) in urine was found to be raised, consistent with findings of carcinoid syndrome. Liver biopsy of the liver lesions confirmed a neuroendocrine tumour.

HOW COMMON IS IT?

- The incidence of all neuroendocrine tumours is 3-5 cases per 100000 population, according to the US surveillance epidemiology and end results database.[2] These tumours are slow growing, and their prevalence is much higher, 35 per 100000 cases[3]
- Carcinoid syndrome occurs in 30-40% of patients with neuroendocrine tumours arising from the small bowel and 5% of those with bronchial neuroendocrine tumours.[4] It develops less commonly in neuroendocrine tumours from other primary sites

How is it diagnosed?

Clinical features

Flushing is the most common symptom, described in 94% of patients in one study.[9] It is characteristically a sudden onset of pink to red discoloration involving the face and upper trunk, lasting for 5-10 minutes and occurring intermittently and at any time throughout the day, but especially during times of stress. Patients may not notice episodes of flushing; it is commonly noted by observers such as family members. Triggers that lead to flushing and diarrhoea include stress, foods containing tyramine (chocolate, walnut, banana, pineapple, tomato, plum, aubergine, avocado), and alcohol. Diarrhoea occurs in 78-84% of patients[9]; urgency is often associated with cramping abdominal pain, occurring both day and night (often irritable bowel syndrome settles at night time). The cramping abdominal pain occurs after large meals in 50% of patients.[9] Symptoms of obstruction are abdominal distension, visible peristalsis, vomiting, or cessation of bowel motions for 1-2 days. Wheezing occurs in 18% of patients and is more common in patients with bronchial neuroendocrine tumours. Other non-specific features include gradual weight loss (30% of cases) and features of right heart failure (seen in 30-40% of cases at presentation).[9]

Investigations

Serotonin secreted in carcinoid syndrome is metabolised to 5-hyroxyindolacetic acid (5-HIAA), which is excreted in the urine and can be measured with a random urine test or a 24 hour urine collection. These tests are >90% sensitive and specific for carcinoid syndrome,[10] although false positives are common if a tyramine-free diet is not adhered to for at least 24 hours before these tests (see http://www.carcinoid.org/pcf/docs/5HIAA.htm).

When there are liver metastases, carcinoid syndrome develops when serotonin reaches the systemic circulation.[11] A general practitioner who suspects carcinoid syndrome should request a urinary 5-HIAA test and abdominal ultrasound (sensitivity 83%) to identify possible metastases.[11] If these are positive or if clinical suspicion is high, refer patients to a gastroenterologist or specialist centre for more definitive diagnosis. Specialised tests may include serum chromogranin A, which is released from neuroendocrine cells; this test is performed at reference laboratories and has a >90% sensitivity.[10] Octreoscan is a nuclear medicine investigation used for staging these tumours; it has a sensitivity of >90% and specificity of 86%.[12 13] Octreoscan and chromogranin A are required for establishing a diagnosis, and octreoscan is helpful for staging disease.

How is it managed?

Symptoms from carcinoid syndrome are managed with somatostatin analogues (octreotide and lanreotide) and interferon alfa, leading to good symptom control in >90% of patients with somatostatin analogues and >80% of patients with interferon alfa.[7] Treatments available for neuroendocrine tumours include surgery, chemotherapy, biotherapy, radiotargeted peptide therapy, and biological agents.[7 11] Surgery is potentially curative, with five year survival of 91-100% at stages 1-3,[14] although the five year survival for patients with distal metastatic disease (stage 4) is 39-50%.[2 5]

Contributors: RS wrote the first draft, which was substantially modified by DS and JKR. RS is guarantor.

Funding: RS, DS, and JKR have support from King's College Hospital and Bexley Care Trust for the submitted work.

Competing interests: All authors have completed the unified competing interest form at www.icmje.org/coi_disclosure.pdf (available on request from the corresponding author) and declare no support from any organisation for the submitted work; no financial relationships with any organisation that might have an interest in the submitted work in the previous three years; and no other relationships or activities that could appear to have influenced the submitted work.

Provenance and peer review: Not commissioned; externally peer reviewed.

1 Kaltsas G, Grossman AB. Clinical features of gastroenteropancreatic tumours. In: Caplin ME, Kvols L, eds. Handbook of neuroendocrine tumours. Bristol: BioScientifica, 2007:53-82.
2 Modlin IM, Lye KD, Kidd M. A 5-decade analysis of 13,715 carcinoid tumors. *Cancer* 2003;97:934-59.
3 Yao JC, Hassan M, Phan A, Dagohoy C, Leary C, Mares JE, et al. One hundred years after "carcinoid": epidemiology of and prognostic factors for neuroendocrine tumors in 35,825 cases in the United States. *J Clin Oncol* 2008;26:3063-72.
4 Ghevariya V, Malieckal A, Ghevariya N, Mazumder M, Anand S. Carcinoid tumors of the gastrointestinal tract. *South Med J* 2009;102:1032-40.
5 Modlin IM, Oberg K, Chung DC, Jensen RT, de Herder WW, Thakker RV, et al. Gastroenteropancreatic neuroendocrine tumours. *Lancet Oncol* 2008;9:61-72.
6 Toth-Fejel S, Pommier RF. Relationships among delay of diagnosis, extent of disease, and survival in patients with abdominal carcinoid tumors. *Am J Surg* 2004;187:575-9.
7 Srirajaskanthan R, Toumpanakis C, Meyer T, Caplin ME. Review article: future therapies for management of metastatic gastroenteropancreatic neuroendocrine tumours. *Aliment Pharmacol Ther* 2009;29:1143-54.
8 Osborne DA, Zervos EE, Strosberg J, Boe BA, Malafa M, Rosemurgy AS, et al. Improved outcome with cytoreduction versus embolization for symptomatic hepatic metastases of carcinoid and neuroendocrine tumors. *Ann Surg Oncol* 2006;13:572-81.
9 Creutzfeldt W. Carcinoid tumors: development of our knowledge. *World J Surg* 1996;20:126-31.
10 De Herder WW. Biochemistry of neuroendocrine tumours. *Best Pract Res Clin Endocrinol Metab* 2007;21:33-41.
11 Ramage JK, Davies AH, Ardill J, Bax N, Caplin M, Grossman A, et al. Guidelines for the management of gastroenteropancreatic neuroendocrine (including carcinoid) tumours. *Gut* 2005;54(suppl 4): 1-16.
12 Gibril F, Reynolds JC, Doppman JL, Chen CC, Venzon DJ, Termanini B, et al. Somatostatin receptor scintigraphy: its sensitivity compared with that of other imaging methods in detecting primary and metastatic gastrinomas. A prospective study. *Ann Intern Med* 1996;125:26-34.
13 Gibril F, Reynolds JC, Chen CC, Yu F, Goebel SU, Serrano J, et al. Specificity of somatostatin receptor scintigraphy: a prospective study and effects of false-positive localizations on management in patients with gastrinomas. *J Nucl Med* 1999;40:539-53.
14 Durante C, Boukheris H, Dromain C, Duvillard P, Leboulleux S, Elias D, et al. Prognostic factors influencing survival from metastatic (stage IV) gastroenteropancreatic well-differentiated endocrine carcinoma. *Endocr Relat Cancer* 2009;16:585-97.

Febrile neutropenia

Jay D Naik, academic clinical lecturer in medical oncology[1],
Suren R K Sathiyaseelan, general practitioner[2],
Naveen S Vasudev, academic clinical lecturer in medical oncology[1]

[1]St James's Institute of Medical Oncology, St James's University Hospital, Leeds LS9 7TF, UK

[2]The Surgery at Nursery Lane and Adel, Leeds LS17 7AQ

Correspondence to: N S Vasudev n.vasudev@leeds.ac.uk

Cite this as: *BMJ* 2010;341:c6981

DOI: 10.1136/bmj.c6981

www.bmj.com/content/341/bmj.c6981

The definition of febrile neutropenia varies but is generally regarded as the presence of a fever >38°C with an absolute neutrophil count of <1.0×10⁹/L. Febrile neutropenia is a result of bone marrow suppression, a common side effect of chemotherapy. Patients with neutropenia are susceptible to developing life threatening bacterial infection. Infection should also be considered in any systemically unwell patient receiving chemotherapy, even if no fever is present.

Why is it missed?

Cases of febrile neutropenia continue to be missed at initial presentation, as medicolegal reports and the 2008 National Confidential Enquiry into Patient Outcome and Death (NCEPOD) show.[5 6 7] National guidance states that all patients receiving chemotherapy should be given both verbal and written information about their treatment, likely side effects, and details of whom to contact if problems arise.[4] Many patients will have access to a dedicated chemotherapy helpline, but this is not universal and not always used.[5] The 2008 national enquiry also found that among patients who became unwell while receiving chemotherapy, only 19% phoned a chemotherapy helpline, 32% contacted their general practitioner, and 41% attended an emergency department as first point of contact.[5]

Cases of febrile neutropenia may be missed because it is not considered.[6 7] Patients may not necessarily volunteer that they are receiving chemotherapy because they may assume that their own doctor knows about their treatment, and doctors handling calls out of hours in primary care centres may not have access to the patient record and may not ask. Finally, the seriousness of febrile neutropenia may not be recognised. An inability to mount an adequate inflammatory response means the signs and symptoms of infection may be minimal, particularly in those receiving corticosteroids. Patients may initially appear well, providing false reassurance to doctors, patients, and carers (case scenario).

Why does this matter?

Even when treated appropriately, febrile neutropenia carries an overall mortality of about 5%.[1 8] Patients can quickly decompensate, and even short delays in treatment can be clinically important. Therefore all patients with a fever who are receiving chemotherapy should be referred immediately for assessment (ideally by their treating oncology team) and an urgent full blood count.

National guidelines state that all patients should receive (intravenous broad spectrum) antibiotics within 60 minutes.[4]

KEY POINTS

- Suspect febrile neutropenia in patients receiving chemotherapy who develop a fever of 38°C or higher or appear systemically unwell
- Remember to ask patients with a recent diagnosis of cancer if they are receiving chemotherapy as they may not always offer this information
- In all cases of suspected febrile neutropenia, refer the patient to hospital (ideally to their treating team) for an urgent full blood count, assessment, and consideration of immediate antibiotic treatment. Do not wait for results of a full blood count test sent from the surgery, as patients may decompensate rapidly

CASE SCENARIO

A 33 year old man presented to his local district hospital a week after chemotherapy, stating that he had a moist cough, with a fever of 38.8 at home. As he had no fever and appeared well on examination, with no abnormal chest findings, he was prescribed amoxicillin and discharged. Over the next 24 hours he became increasingly unwell and presented at the emergency department with septic shock and severe neutropenia (neutrophils 0.02×10^9/L). Despite fluids and broad spectrum antibiotics, the patient died.

HOW COMMON IS FEBRILE NEUTROPENIA?

- The risk of febrile neutropenia varies widely (5%-50%) depending on the chemotherapy regimen[1 2 3]
- The number of patients receiving chemotherapy each year in England is increasing[4]
- An estimated 65 000 chemotherapy programmes (a planned period of repeated cycles of treatment) are delivered annually in England.[4] On the basis of this figure, we conservatively estimate that at least 10 000 episodes of febrile neutropenia occur annually
- Risk increases with age (65 years and over), advanced stage of disease, presence of comorbidities, haematological malignancy, and absence of haematopoietic colony-stimulating factors support, and if a patient has had a previous episode of febrile neutropenia[3]

How is it diagnosed?

Clinical

The diagnosis of febrile neutropenia in primary care is a clinical one and requires general practitioners to be vigilant. Specifically ask patients with a recent diagnosis of cancer if they have recently had chemotherapy. Remember that haematological malignancies can cause myelosuppression in patients who have not received treatment. Timing may give guidance on a patient's risk of being neutropenic—for example, in patients with solid malignancies receiving chemotherapy every three weeks, the risk of neutropenia is typically greatest from day 7 to day 14. However, timing is often unpredictable and should not therefore be relied on.

Patients' symptoms are often non-specific with no localising features. Symptoms may include feeling hot or cold, rigors, sweats, influenza-like symptoms, and general malaise. Ask about sore mouth and diarrhoea, which also commonly occur after chemotherapy, as mucositis can be a portal of entry for host flora into the bloodstream.

Clinical examination should aim to establish quickly how unwell the patient is. Check the temperature and specifically look for signs of shock. This is more likely in patients with dyspnoea, dehydration, diarrhoea, and altered mental state.[9] Look for a focus of infection, although this is often not apparent. In patients with indwelling central venous lines, check the subcutaneous portion of the line and its exit site for signs of infection. Ask specifically about rigors associated with flushing the line as this may also indicate an infection associated with the line.

Investigations

If febrile neutropenia is suspected, refer the patient immediately to hospital (ideally to his or her treating team) for an urgent full blood count, where appropriate cultures, other blood tests, and radiological investigations can also be performed.

How is it managed?

Primary care doctors should ideally discuss patients with the treating department if they have any concerns about the management of unwell patients receiving chemotherapy. After admission to hospital, empiric broad spectrum intravenous antibiotics, according to the local policy on febrile neutropenia, should be promptly administered. This should be done before the full blood count result is known if the patient is in shock. Additional supportive measures, such as administration of intravenous fluids, may be necessary initially. The use of colony stimulating factors can be considered in patients at high risk, such as with expected prolonged (>10 days) or profound (<0.1×10^9/L) neutropenia, hypotension, and multiorgan failure.[1] Stratification tools are sometimes used in secondary care to identify patients at low risk who can be treated safely with oral antibiotics in hospital with subsequent early discharge.[10]

Contributors: JDN had the original idea for the paper. NSV wrote the first draft and all authors contributed to the final draft. NSV is the guarantor.

Funding: No special funding.

Competing interests: All authors have completed the Unified Competing Interest form at www.icmje.org/coi_disclosure.pdf (available on request from the corresponding author) (URL) and declare: no financial support for the submitted work from anyone other than their employer; no financial relationships with commercial entities that might have an interest in the submitted work; no spouses, partners, or children with relationships with commercial entities that might have an interest in the submitted work; no non-financial interests that may be relevant to the submitted work.

Provenance and peer review: Not commissioned; externally peer reviewed.

Patient consent not required (patient anonymised, dead, or hypothetical).

1 Smith TJ, Khatcheressian J, Lyman GH, Ozer H, Armitage JO, Balducci L, et al. 2006 update of recommendations for the use of white blood cell growth factors: an evidence-based clinical practice guideline. *J Clin Oncol* 2006;24:3187-205.
2 Kuderer NM, Dale DC, Crawford J, Lyman GH. Impact of primary prophylaxis with granulocyte colony-stimulating factor on febrile neutropenia and mortality in adult cancer patients receiving chemotherapy: a systematic review. *J Clin Oncol* 2007;25:3158-67.
3 Aapro MS, Cameron DA, Pettengell R, Bohilus J, Crawford J, Ellis M, et al. EORTC guidelines for the use of granulocyte-colony stimulating factor to reduce the incidence of chemotherapy-induced febrile neutropenia in adult patients with lymphomas and solid tumours. *Eur J Cancer* 2006;42:2433-53.
4 National Chemotherapy Advisory Group. Chemotherapy services in England: ensuring quality and safety. 2009. www.dh.gov.uk/en/Publicationsandstatistics/Publications/DH_104500.
5 National Confidentional Enquiry into Patient Outcome and Death. For better, for worse? 2008. www.ncepod.org.uk.
6 Medical Protection Society. A false reassurance. *Casebook* 2010;18(2):19. www.medicalprotection.org/uk/case-reports-may-2010/a-false-reassurance.
7 Medical Protection Society. Sepsis following chemotherapy. *Casebook* 2003;11(4):20www.medicalprotection.org/uk/casebook/november2003/case-reports/sepsis-following-chemotherapy.
8 De Naurois J, Novitzky-Basso I, Gill MJ, Marti FM, Cullen MH, Roila F, et al. Management of febrile neutropenia: ESMO clinical practice guidelines. *Ann Oncol* 2010;21(suppl 5):v252-6.
9 Malik I, Hussain M, Yousuf H. Clinical characteristics and therapeutic outcome of patients with febrile neutropenia who present in shock: need for better strategies. *J Infect* 2001;42:120-35.
10 Klastersky J, Paesmans M, Rubenstein EB, Boyer M, Elting L, Feld R, et al. The Multinational Association for Supportive Care in Cancer risk index: a multinational scoring system for identifying low-risk febrile neutropenic cancer patients. *J Clin Oncol* 2000;18:3038-51.

Primary HIV infection

Gautam Das, specialist registrar,
Piero Baglioni, consultant physician,
Onyebuchi Okosieme, consultant physician

Prince Charles Hospital, Gurnos, Merthyr Tydfil CF47 9DT

Correspondence to: G Das drgdas@gmail.com

Cite this as: *BMJ* 2010;341:c4583

DOI: 10.1136/bmj.c4583

www.bmj.com/content/341/bmj.c4583

Primary HIV infection encompasses the biological and clinical manifestations of the period between initial contact with the virus and the appearance of specific antibodies.[1]

Why is primary HIV infection missed?

Primary HIV infection is symptomatic in most individuals but is easy to miss.[3 4] In a cohort study of 46 patients with primary HIV infection, only a quarter of those with acute presentations caused by primary HIV infection were correctly diagnosed in various acute and primary care settings in the United States.[5] The diagnosis of primary HIV infection was also missed at initial presentation in 19 of 40 patients (48%) in the United Kingdom.[3] The infection may be missed because the symptoms are transient, often lasting less than two weeks, and tend to overlap with those of infections that are much more common in clinical practice. Failure to elicit a history of exposure to the virus, reluctance to test, and lack of awareness of the limitations of testing in the acute phase may also contribute to diagnostic delay.[3 4]

Why does this matter?

The diagnosis of primary HIV infection has individual and public health benefits. If the infection is not recognised, a clinically silent phase follows, during which CD4 T lymphocyte counts gradually decline.[1] Early diagnosis allows monitoring for the onset of immunodeficiency and timely institution of highly active antiretroviral treatment. Late diagnosis is associated with HIV related morbidity and mortality and adds to the cost of treatment.[6] Patients with primary HIV infection have high levels of viraemia and are more likely to transmit the infection by sexual contact.[1] Counselling may thus reduce sexual risk behaviours and transmission of infection.[7]

How is it diagnosed?

Clinical features

Fever is the most common symptom, present in 80-90% of patients. It typically appears two to four weeks after the infection and is commonly associated with sore throat and cervical lymphadenopathy. This may lead to the erroneous diagnosis of mononucleosis or tonsillitis.[5] A non-specific maculopapular rash is seen in over 40% of patients but may be difficult to detect in patients with darkly pigmented skin.[1] Headache may be present in over 50% of patients and may suggest HIV invasion of the central nervous system, an early event in the natural course of the infection.[5] Primary HIV infection must be included in the differential diagnosis of patients presenting with aseptic meningitis.[8]

KEY POINTS

- Primary HIV infection should be suspected in people at risk of HIV who present with an acute viral illness
- Diagnosis of primary HIV infection may reduce HIV transmission through modification of sexual risk behaviour and will allow monitoring for immune deficiency and timely institution of highly active antiretroviral treatment when indicated
- First line testing comprises both HIV antibody and p24 antigen levels
- If a patient declines testing, explore and document the reasons for this, correcting any inaccurate beliefs

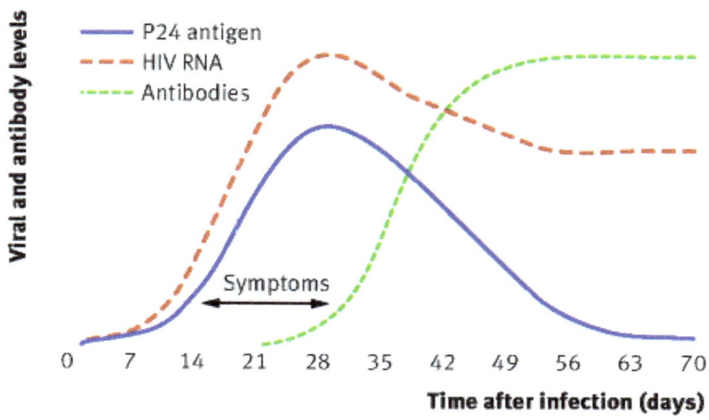

Fig 1 Approximate time course of viral and antibody changes during primary HIV infection

Diagnosis is easier if the patient volunteers the information of possible exposure to HIV or is known to belong to a high risk group for the disease. Disclosing this information may, however, be difficult both for the patient and the doctor (case scenario) owing to the need to probe into the sensitive issues surrounding HIV, such as high risk sexual behaviour and substance misuse. These difficulties can be magnified when clinical contact is occasional and there is little time to forge a close doctor-patient relationship. If a patient refuses a test, explore the reasons for this and correct any inaccurate beliefs about infection or the consequences of testing; document the patient's reasons for declining the test.[9]

In developed countries, men having sex with men represent the category most at risk of primary HIV infection. Unprotected anal (less commonly oral) intercourse remains the primary route for transmission.[10] Most heterosexual patients with HIV in the United Kingdom have contracted the disease abroad, mostly in sub-Saharan Africa.[10] However, the number of people infected heterosexually in the UK is increasing. Transmission through injecting drug use and mother to child transmission have remained low since the start of the epidemic.[2]

Investigations

By definition, primary HIV infection precedes seroconversion, and therefore testing limited to viral antibodies may initially convey negative or borderline results.[1] The infection is characterised by a high plasma virus load, and direct testing for viral antigen (p24 antigen) or nucleic acid (HIV RNA) usually confirms the diagnosis (tture).[1] Although p24 antigen testing is less sensitive than HIV RNA (88.7% *v* 100%), it is usually preferred in non-specialist settings because it is less expensive (£2 *v* £75 in our institution) and associated with fewer false positive results (100% *v* 97.4% specificity).[11]

Nowadays testing for antibodies and p24 antigen can be carried out simultaneously, and clinicians should liaise with local laboratories about available tests. As highlighted in a recent statement by the British Association of Sexual Health and HIV (BASHH), patients presenting very early after onset of symptoms may still be missed by currently available tests. When such tests first give negative results, follow-up testing is recommended three months later.[12] Antibodies are detectable three to 12 weeks after infection but may occasionally take as long as six to 12 months to appear.[1] Pretest counselling does not usually need to be lengthy but should cover the benefits of testing and how the results will be conveyed. Written consent is also not routinely necessary as this may discourage the test by according it special status.[9]

How is it managed?

After diagnosis, refer the patient immediately to a specialist for further investigation and management.[9] Results should be clearly communicated in person and in a confidential environment. Avoid detailed counselling after HIV testing but reassure the patient that their symptoms are temporary and do not reflect permanent immunosuppression and that the condition is treatable.[1 9] Also explore available support to the patient for coping with the diagnosis. Finally, discuss appropriate measures to prevent onward transmission of infection.

CASE SCENARIO

A previously healthy 19 year old man was admitted to our medical ward with a history of fever, sore throat, and a maculopapular rash on his trunk. An upper respiratory tract infection had been diagnosed in the community a few days before. A monospot test (for infectious mononucleosis caused by Epstein-Barr virus) was negative, and he initially denied risky sexual behaviour and declined an offer of HIV testing. His symptoms improved, but before discharge he mentioned to the ward sister that he had had a casual sexual encounter with a man a few weeks earlier. He then consented to an HIV test, which was positive for the p24 antigen.

HOW COMMON IS PRIMARY HIV INFECTION?[2]

- Symptoms are present in 50-90% of individuals with primary HIV infection[1]
- During 2008 there were 7298 new diagnoses of HIV in the United Kingdom. In the same year, 27% of the estimated 83000 people with HIV were thought to be unaware of their infection (because many people only realise they have HIV infection when they develop full blown AIDS)
- The two groups with the highest HIV prevalence in the UK are men who have sex with men, and black African heterosexuals. The number of new infections acquired heterosexually increased by 53% (from 740 to 1130 cases) from 2004 to 2008
- The estimated numbers of new infections acquired through injecting drug use and mother to child transmission (170 and 110 cases respectively in 2008) have remained stable since the start of the epidemic

Contributors: PB had the original idea for the paper. GD wrote the first draft and all authors contributed to the final draft. OO is the guarantor.

Funding: No special funding.

Competing interests: All authors have completed the Unified Competing Interest form at http://www.icmje.org/coi_disclosure.pdf (available on request from the corresponding author) and declare no support from any company for the submitted work; no authors have any relationships with companies that might have an interest in the submitted work in the previous three years; their spouses, partners, or children have no financial relationships that may be relevant to the submitted work; and all authors have no non-financial interests that may be relevant to the submitted work.

Provenance and peer review: Not commissioned; externally peer reviewed.

Patient consent obtained.

1 Kassutto S, Rosenberg ES. Primary HIV type 1 infection. *Clin Infect Dis* 2004;38:1447-53.
2 Health Protection Agency. *HIV in the United Kingdom: 2009 report.* 2009. www.hpa.org.uk/web/HPAweb&HPAwebStandard/HPAweb_C/1259151891866.
3 Sudarshi D, Pao D, Murphy G, Parry J, Dean G, Fisher M. Missed opportunities for diagnosing primary HIV infection. *Sex Transm Infect* 2008;84:14-6.
4 Weintrob AC, Giner J, Menezes P, Patrick E, Benjamin DK Jr, Lennox J, et al. Infrequent diagnosis of primary human immunodeficiency virus infection: missed opportunities in acute care settings. *Arch Intern Med* 2003;163:2097-100.
5 Schacker T, Collier AC, Hughes J, Shea T, Corey L. Clinical and epidemiological features of primary HIV infection. *Ann Intern Med* 1996;125:257-64.
6 Kitahata MM, Gange SJ, Abraham AG, Merriman B, Saag MS, Justice AC, et al. Effect of early versus deferred antiretroviral therapy for HIV on survival. *N Engl J Med* 2009;360:1815-26.
7 Koblin BA. Effect of behavioural intervention to reduce acquisition of HIV infection among men who have sex with men: the EXPLORE randomised control study. *Lancet* 2004;364:41-50.
8 Newton PJ, Newsholme W, Brink NS, Manji H, Williams IG, Miller RF. Acute meningoencephalitis and meningitis due to primary HIV infection. *BMJ* 2002;325:1225-7.
9 British HIV Asscociation. UK national guidelines for HIV testing 2008. www.bhiva.org/HIVTesting2008.aspx.
10 Macdonald N, Elam G, Hickson F, Imrie J, McGarrigle CA, Fenton KA, et al. Factors associated with HIV seroconversion in gay men in England at the start of the 21st century. *Sex Transm Infect* 2008;84:8-13.
11 Daar ES, Little S, Pitt J, Santangelo J, Ho P, Harawa N, et al. Diagnosis of primary HIV-1 infection. *Ann Intern Med* 2001;134:25-9.
12 British Association of Sexual Health and HIV. *BASHH statement on HIV window period: March 2010.* 2010. www.bashh.org/guidelines.

Infective endocarditis

Mark Connaughton, consultant cardiologist[1],
John G Rivett, general practitioner[2]

[1]Cardiology Department, St Mary's Hospital, Newport, Isle of Wight PO30 5TG, UK

[2]Martins Oak Surgery, Battle TN33 0EA UK

Correspondence to: M Connaughton mark.connaughton@iow.nhs.uk

Cite this as: *BMJ* 2010;341:c6596

DOI: 10.1136/bmj.c6596

www.bmj.com/content/341/bmj.c6596

Infective endocarditis is caused by microbial infection of the endocardial surface or of prosthetic material in the heart. More than 80% of cases are caused by *Staphylococcus aureus* or by species of *Streptococcus* or *Enterococcus*. The total incidence of infective endocarditis has remained relatively constant, but the epidemiology has changed markedly in recent years. Proportionately more cases are now seen in association with prosthetic valves and as a result of hospital acquired infections.[1]

Why is infective endocarditis missed?

Infective endocarditis is a rare disease with varied presentations. Symptoms such as loss of appetite, weight loss, arthralgia, and night sweats overlap with much more common conditions, including occult malignancy. Fever is almost invariable,[2] but many patients may initially experience only a general malaise. Given the diagnostic difficulty, some 25% of patients take longer than one month to be admitted to hospital after their first clinical signs become evident.[2]

Why does this matter?

Data from the pre-antibiotic era suggest that infective endocarditis is almost always fatal if untreated.[3] Delayed diagnosis in some groups is associated with a substantial increase in mortality.[4] Even with timely recognition and treatment, the outcome may sometimes be poor. Observational studies report one year mortality of 20-25% and 10 year mortality of 50%, outcomes worse than for many malignancies.[5]

How is it diagnosed?

Infective endocarditis should remain part of the differential diagnosis of a persistent febrile or inflammatory illness. Ironically, once infective endocarditis is suspected, confirmation of the diagnosis may be straightforward. This will usually involve referral to secondary care, where modified Duke criteria (box 1) may be applied as the diagnostic standard. These use a synthesis of clinical, microbiological, and echocardiographic findings.[6] The negative predictive value of these criteria has been estimated as more than 92%.[7] So called "culture negative" endocarditis, which occurs in 20-30% of cases, remains a difficult challenge and may be underdiagnosed by Duke criteria.[8]

The NHS Map of Medicine suggests an algorithm for early diagnosis (http://eng.mapofmedicine.com/evidence/map/infective_endocarditis3.html) but anticipates this as taking place exclusively in secondary care.

KEY POINTS

- Infective endocarditis is rare but is fatal in about a fifth of cases
- Infective endocarditis should be part of the differential diagnosis of a persistent febrile or inflammatory illness, particularly if there are pre-existing cardiac lesions
- Diagnosis usually requires consistent clinical findings, positive blood cultures, or other proof of infection, and positive echocardiographic findings
- Treatment is prolonged and may require cardiac surgery in addition to an extended course of antibiotics

BOX 1 DUKE CRITERIA FOR DIAGNOSIS OF ENDOCARDITIS*

Requirements for diagnosis of "definite" infective endocarditis†

Pathological criteria

- Histological diagnosis from tissue, or culture of tissue or intracardiac abscess

Clinical criteria

- Two major criteria or
- One major criterion and three minor criteria or
- Five minor criteria

Requirements for diagnosis of "possible" infective endocarditis

Clinical criteria

- One major criterion and one minor criterion or
- Three minor criteria

Rejection of infective endocarditis if one of the following conditions is met

- Firm, alternative diagnosis explaining the evidence suggesting infective endocarditis
- Resolution of clinical findings of infective endocarditis with antibiotic course lasting four days or less
- No pathological evidence of infective endocarditis at surgery or autopsy with antibiotic course lasting four days or less
- The condition does not meet criteria for "definite" or "possible" infective endocarditis

Major blood culture criteria

- Two positive blood cultures for typical infective endocarditis organisms
- Persistently positive cultures for such organisms taken >12 hours apart
- Three or more positive cultures taken at least one hour apart

Major echocardiographic criteria

- Echocardiogram indicating infective endocarditis with no alternative explanation
- Myocardial abscess
- New partial dehiscence of prosthetic valve
- New valvular regurgitation

Minor criteria

- Predisposing cardiac condition
- Intravenous drug use
- Fever (≥38°C)
- Raised C reactive protein or erythrocyte sedimentation rate
- Vascular lesions including major arterial emboli, septic pulmonary infarcts, mycotic aneurysm, intracranial haemorrhage, conjunctival haemorrhages, and Janeway lesions
- Immunological phenomena, including glomerulonephritis, Roth spots, Osler's nodes, and positive rheumatoid factor
- Positive cultures not meeting a major criterion or serological evidence of active infection with an organism consistent with infective endocarditis
- Echocardiographic results consistent with infective endocarditis but not meeting a major criterion

**Adapted from the American Heart Association[6]*

†Either the pathological or the clinical criteria need to be met

BOX 2 RISK FACTORS (AND PREVALENCE) FOUND IN PATIENTS IN EUROPE WHO WERE SUBSEQUENTLY DIAGNOSED WITH "DEFINITE" ENDOCARDITIS ACCORDING TO DUKE CRITERIA[2]

- Predisposing native valve condition (31%)
- Invasive procedure within previous 60 days (25%)
- Prosthetic valve (20%)
- Presence of pacemaker (12%)
- Congenital heart disease (10%)
- Current intravenous drug use (9%)
- Previous endocarditis (7%)

Clinical features

Pre-existing risk factors for infective endocarditis (box 2) should arouse suspicion, but previously well individuals can also become infected. In one series of endocarditis *S aureus*, only 55% of patients had a pre-existing valve lesion and 68% of patients did not show a portal of entry.[8] A fever >38ćC at some point is almost invariable,[2] so the absence of any fever should lead to consideration of an alternative diagnosis. Diagnostic "red flags" include a new regurgitant murmur, which is found in almost half of patients[2]; a regurgitant murmur across a prosthetic valve; and any systemic embolus or sepsis of unknown origin.[9] In primary care, the combination of the failure of a febrile illness to resolve, together with a murmur, may be "as good as it gets" in terms of early clinical indicators. Painless Janeway lesions on the palms or soles and immunological findings such as Roth spots and Osler nodes are now rare, being found in no more than 5% of cases of infective endocarditis,[2] but they are useful if they are present and recognised.

Investigations

A definitive diagnosis of infective endocarditis will almost certainly require referral to secondary care. Initial testing in primary care may prompt earlier referral or, conversely, provide reassurance that an inflammatory condition seems to be settling. Although markers of inflammation such as erythrocyte sedimentation rate and C reactive protein are raised in over 60% of patients with infective endocarditis,[2] these tests alone are too non-discriminatory to make or exclude the diagnosis.[10] However, raised concentrations (considered to be minor Duke criteria) may aid a decision to refer. A positive rheumatoid factor is potentially useful as a minor criterion. Positive blood cultures for *S aureus*, *Streptococcus*, or *Enterococcus* species suggest an important infection in any context and should be referred for hospital assessment.

Positive blood cultures or other serology and cardiac imaging in secondary care are the mainstays of definitive diagnosis. Transthoracic echocardiography is readily available, but transoesophageal studies are the current best imaging modality, particularly if prosthetic material is present. Specificity for detecting vegetations, abscesses, or other evidence of infective endocarditis can approach 100%.[11] Serial studies should be performed if the initial diagnosis remains in doubt.

How is it managed?

Hospital care is mandatory for at least the initial treatment of infective endocarditis in order to assess the early response to antibiotics and to monitor and treat any complications. Little controlled trial evidence exists to guide treatment, but a substantial body of clinical experience does exist.[6 9] Rational management involves extended courses of high dose antibiotic treatment, ideally guided by microbiological sensitivity testing. In one series of over 200 patients, 38% of patients needed surgical treatment.[5] Indications for surgery include failure to control the infection, threatened or actual embolus of septic material, and development of heart failure. Some patients may be suitable for outpatient intravenous

CASE SCENARIO

Four months after prostate surgery that had been complicated by a urinary infection, a 65 year old man presented with lethargy, malaise, and mild anaemia. No further specific abnormalities were found over the next two weeks. He developed night sweats, and a new systolic murmur was heard. C reactive protein was raised at 90 mg/l. Infective endocarditis was considered as a diagnosis. Blood cultures were ordered and he was referred to hospital. *Enterococcus faecalis* was grown from all culture bottles. Transthoracic echocardiography showed mitral valve vegetations, confirming the diagnosis of bacterial endocarditis.

HOW COMMON IS INFECTIVE ENDOCARDITIS?

- The annual incidence is 3-10 cases per 100000
- A general practitioner is unlikely to see more than one case every 8-10 years

antibiotic treatment after an initial inpatient assessment and treatment period.[9] After discharge from hospital, patients need monitoring for relapse or recurrent infection. Patients remain at risk of further episodes of infective endocarditis and should be counselled to report any potentially relevant symptoms.

Contributors: MC was the main author of this article and JGR contributed. MC will act as guarantor.

Competing interests: All authors have completed the Unified Competing Interest form at www.icmje.org/coi_disclosure.pdf (available on request from the corresponding author) and declare that they have no relationships with any companies that might have an interest in the submitted work in the previous 3 years; their spouses, partners, or children have no financial relationships that may be relevant to the submitted work; and the authors have no non-financial interests that may be relevant to the submitted work.

Provenance and peer review: Commissioned; externally peer reviewed.

Patient consent not required (patient anonymised, dead, or hypothetical).

1 Hill EE, Herijgers P, Herregods M-C, Peetermans WE. Evolving trends in infective endocarditis. *Clin Micobiol Infect* 2006;12:5-12.
2 Murdoch DR, Corey GR, Hoen B, Miró JM, Fowler VG Jr, Bayer AS, et al. Clinical presentation, etiology, and outcome of infective endocarditis in the 21st century: the International Collaboration on Endocarditis—Prospective Cohort Study. *Arch Intern Med* 2009;169:463-73.
3 Verhagen DWM, Vedder AC, Speelman P, van der Meer JTM. Antimicrobial treatment of infective endocarditis caused by viridans streptococci highly susceptible to penicillin: historic overview and future considerations. *J Antimicrob Chemother* 2006;57:819-24.
4 San Martin J, Sarriá C, de las Cuevas C, Duarte J, Gamallo C. Relevance of clinical presentation and period of diagnosis in prosthetic valve endocarditis. *J Heart Valve Dis* 2010;19:131-8.
5 Netzer ROM, Altwegg SC, Zollinger E, Tauber M, Carrel T, Seiler C. Infective endocarditis: determinants of long term outcome. *Heart* 2002;88:61-6.
6 American Heart Association. Scientific statement. Infective endocarditis. Diagnosis, antimicrobial therapy and management of complications. *Circulation* 2005;111:e394-434.
7 Dodds GA, Sexton DJ, Durack DT, Bashore TM, Corey GR, Kisslo J. Negative predictive value of the Duke criteria for infective endocarditis. *Am J Cardiol* 1996;77:403-7.
8 Hill EE, Vanderschueren, S, Verhaegen J, Herijgers P, Claus P, Herregods M-C, et al. Risk factors for infective endocarditis and outcome of patients with Staphylococcus aureus bacteremia. *Mayo Clinic Proc* 2007;82:1165-9.
9 Task Force on the Prevention, Diagnosis, and Treatment of Infective Endocarditis of the European Society of Cardiology (ESC). Guidelines on the prevention, diagnosis, and treatment of infective endocarditis (new version 2009). *Eur Heart J* 2009;30:2369-413.
10 Gouriet F, Botelho-Nevers E, Coulibaly, B, Raoult D, Casalta JP. Evaluation of Sedimentation rate, rheumatoid factor, C-reactive protein, and tumor necrosis factor for the diagnosis of infective endocarditis. *Clin Vaccine Immunol* 2006;13:301.
11 Rozich JD, Edwards WD, Hanna RD. Mechanical prosthetic valve-associated strands: pathologic correlates to transesophageal echocardiography. *J Am Soc Echocardiogr* 2003;16:97-100.

Imported malaria

Merlin L Willcox, general practitioner[1],
Jill Mant, paediatric specialist registrar[2],
Tim O'Dempsey, consultant in tropical medicine[3]

[1]Department of Primary Care Health Sciences, University of Oxford, Oxford OX1 2EP, UK

[2]Department of Paediatrics, Luton Hospital, Luton, UK

[3]Liverpool School of Tropical Medicine, Liverpool, UK

Correspondence to: M L Willcox merlin.willcox@phc.ox.ac.uk

Cite this as: *BMJ* 2013;346:f3214

DOI: 10.1136/bmj.f3214

www.bmj.com/content/346/bmj.f3214

A 19 year old student phoned an official health service telephone helpline with a 10 day history of aching legs, vomiting, diarrhoea, and abdominal pain. She mentioned a recent trip to Uganda but was reassured and told she had "flu." The next day her boyfriend took her to see her doctor, where she mentioned general malaise, tiredness, and occasional nausea; the doctor diagnosed a viral illness and advised her to keep taking paracetamol. Three days later a friend found her dead in bed in her university halls of residence. The coroner recorded death due to cerebral malaria.[1]

What is malaria?

Malaria is an infection caused by protozoa of the genus *Plasmodium*. Five species infect humans (*P falciparum, P vivax, P ovale, P malariae*, and *P knowlesi*). Most of the fatal cases are caused by *P falciparum*.

Why is malaria missed in non-endemic countries?

As illustrated by the case described here, the symptoms of malaria are non-specific and can easily be mistaken for a viral illness such as influenza, unless clinicians think to ask patients whether they have travelled abroad.

A retrospective observational study of 191 deaths due to malaria in the United Kingdom from 1987 to 2006 found that the case fatality was inversely related to incidence, suggesting that cases were more easily missed by clinicians unaccustomed to seeing this disease.[4] A retrospective series of 39 cases of malaria diagnosed in Sheffield from 2000 to 2005 found that eight of these patients had presented to health professionals with symptoms of malaria but were not immediately referred to hospital or for a diagnostic test, suggesting that the diagnosis of malaria had not been considered.[6] A retrospective case review of 211 children admitted to hospital with malaria in east London found that 114 had initially presented to their doctor, but malaria was suspected at the first visit in only 32% of these, and diagnosis was delayed in 53%, by one to 14 days.[7]

Why does this matter?

If untreated, malaria can be rapidly fatal, particularly in non-immune patients. Delay in diagnosis is associated with an increased risk of severe malaria and death.[5 8] The overall case fatality rate from malaria in the United Kingdom is 0.73%,[4] but for cases with signs of severe malaria (box) this may reach 10-20%.[9] Severe complications and death may occur within 24-48 hours of onset of symptoms.[10 11] Early diagnosis and appropriate treatment are therefore crucial.

KEY POINTS

- If patients have fever, history of fever, or flu-like symptoms, always ask about travel to a malaria endemic country within the past year
- If malaria is suspected, request urgent thick and thin malaria films (three negative films results on consecutive days are needed to exclude the diagnosis) and a full blood count (thrombocytopaenia is common in acute malaria)
- If there are any signs of severe malaria, admit as an emergency

How is malaria diagnosed?

Clinical

Question anyone presenting with a history of fever or flu-like symptoms about travel to malaria endemic countries within the past year. Investigate urgently those returning from a malaria endemic area, regardless of whether they have taken malaria prophylaxis. Intermittent fever may be a feature of malaria, so temperature may be normal at the time of examination. A case series of 482 patients in the United States found that half of adult patients were not febrile when they presented, although most had a history of fever.[12] Other common symptoms include vomiting, diarrhoea, headache, and myalgia.[5 12] Most patients with *P falciparum* present within six months of returning from abroad, although later presentations may occur. The box shows the features of severe disease.

Investigations

It is preferable to refer all patients with suspected malaria to hospital immediately for further investigation because of the risk of rapid progression of falciparum malaria. However, if the patient is relatively well and it is possible to obtain results rapidly (the same day), it may be reasonable to investigate in a primary care setting. This calls for some clinical judgment. If the risk of malaria is low and the patient is not severely ill, outpatient testing with next day results may be acceptable, but the patient should then be advised to reconsult rapidly if there is any worsening of symptoms.

The clinician should request an urgent full blood count and "malaria thick and thin films" (both on the same EDTA sample). Although microscopy is the standard diagnostic method, low density infection may be missed,[13] particularly if microscopists are inexperienced or if patients have taken an antimalarial or an antibiotic with antimalarial activity. Therefore, if the first slide gives a negative result, films should be repeated after 12-24 hours, and again after another 24 hours. The likelihood of malaria is low if experienced microscopists find three consecutive negative blood film results.[14]

In the United Kingdom some haematology laboratories may also be able to perform a rapid diagnostic test. These tests are based on detection of parasite antigens or enzymes; a recent Cochrane review found that the sensitivity and specificity of the most common rapid diagnostic tests were both 95%, compared with microscopy.[15] Rapid diagnostic tests are useful in increasing speed of diagnosis, even in non-endemic countries[16] and, if available, can be used as an adjunct to microscopy, although they cannot replace it. All positive malaria test results should be telephoned immediately to the requesting doctor and communicated by the doctor to the patient.[14]

Thrombocytopenia is common in acute malaria, and, if otherwise unexplained, may be an important clue even if the blood film has been reported as negative. A prospective study looking at returning travellers with fever found that leucocyte counts $<10\times10^9$/L, platelet counts $<150\times10^9$/L, and haemoglobin levels <120 g/L were all associated with an increased probability of malaria. Thrombocytopenia was the best predictor, with a positive likelihood ratio of 11.[17]

How is malaria managed?

Seek expert advice on treatment, particularly if there are signs of complications. In the primary care setting, if there are any signs of severe malaria, refer the patient to hospital as an emergency and treat any complications (for example, shock, hypoglycaemia, convulsions) while awaiting transfer.

Most patients with falciparum malaria need admission to hospital, although recent evidence has suggested that a small selected group with uncomplicated falciparum malaria can be treated safely as outpatients.[18 19] Those with uncomplicated non-falciparum infections can usually be managed as outpatients provided they are able to take oral drugs. Mixed infections can occur and *P falciparum* may be missed or misdiagnosed. Therefore it is sensible to have a low threshold for admission and to advise all those treated as outpatients

HOW COMMON IS MALARIA?

- Worldwide over 200 million cases of malaria occur annually and 0.5-1 million deaths, 90% of which are among children in Africa[2]
- *Plasmodium falciparum* accounted for about 70% of the 1677 cases notified in the United Kingdom in 2011, whereas 25% of cases were due to *P vivax*[3]
- Of the 191 deaths from malaria in the United Kingdom from 1987 to 2006, 184 were due to *P falciparum*[4]
- About 20% of imported malaria cases are in children[5]

DEFINITION OF SEVERE MALARIA[9]

In patients with *Plasmodium falciparum* asexual parasitaemia and no other obvious cause of symptoms, severe malaria is defined by one or more of the following features:

Clinical features

- Impaired consciousness or coma from which patients cannot be roused
- Prostration—that is, generalised weakness such that that patients cannot sit up unaided
- Failure to feed
- Multiple convulsions—more than two episodes in 24 hours
- Deep breathing, respiratory distress (acidotic breathing)
- Circulatory collapse or shock, systolic blood pressure <70 mm Hg in adults and <50 mm Hg in children
- Clinical jaundice plus evidence of other vital organ dysfunction
- Haemoglobinuria
- Abnormal spontaneous bleeding
- Pulmonary oedema (radiological)

Laboratory findings

Haematology

- Severe normocytic anaemia (haemoglobin level <50 g/L, packed cell volume <15%)
- Hyperparasitaemia (>2% or 100 000/µL in areas of low intensity of transmission; >5% or 250 000/µL in areas of high and stable intensity of transmission)

Biochemistry

- Hypoglycaemia (blood glucose level <2.2 mmol/L or <40 mg/dL)
- Renal impairment (serum creatinine level >265 µmol/L)
- Metabolic acidosis (plasma bicarbonate level <15 mmol/L)
- Hyperlactataemia (lactate >5 mmol/L)

Urine

- Haemoglobinuria

to seek further medical attention urgently if they deteriorate. It is also advisable to review all patients with malaria 1-2 weeks after completion of treatment.[18 19]

Because of the risk of increasing drug resistance, the World Health Organization now recommends that uncomplicated *P falciparum* malaria should be treated with artemisinin combination therapies.[9] Recent studies have proved that intravenous artesunate is more effective than quinine for the treatment of severe malaria,[20 21] but UK guidelines still recommend quinine because artesunate is unlicensed in the European Union.[14] These guidelines are, however, currently under review. Chloroquine is usually effective for non-falciparum malarias; however, chloroquine resistant *P vivax* is increasingly prevalent in some areas (for example, Indonesia, Peru, and Oceania).[9] In addition, patients with *P vivax* or *P ovale* infections should have their glucose 6 phosphate dehydrogenase (G6PD) status checked and, unless significantly G6PD deficient, should also be treated with an appropriate course of primaquine to reduce the likelihood of relapses.[22]

UK guidelines for malaria treatment[14] and a useful management algorithm are available at www.hpa.org.uk/Topics/InfectiousDiseases/InfectionsAZ/Malaria/Guidelines/mala20guidelinesTreatment/.

Contributors: MW wrote the first draft of the article, which was revised by the coauthors. All authors read and approved the final manuscript. MW is guarantor of the paper.

Competing interests: All authors have completed the ICMJE uniform disclosure form at http://www.icmje.org/coi_disclosure.pdf (available on request from the corresponding author) and declare: no support from any organisation for the submitted work; no financial relationships with any organisations that might have an interest in the submitted work in the previous three years, no other relationships or activities that could appear to have influenced the submitted work.

Provenance and peer review: Not commissioned; externally peer reviewed.

Patient consent not required (patient anonymised, dead, or hypothetical).

1 Anon. Student died of Malaria after being diagnosed with flu. Secondary student died of malaria after being diagnosed with flu. *Mail Online* 2007 Jan 10. www.dailymail.co.uk/news/article-427932/Student-died-Malaria-diagnosed-flu.html#.

2 World Health Organization. World malaria report 2011. WHO, 2011.

3 Health Protection Agency. Imported malaria cases and deaths, United Kingdom: 1992-2011. Secondary imported malaria cases and deaths, United Kingdom: 1992-2011. 2012. www.hpa.org.uk/Topics/InfectiousDiseases/InfectionsAZ/Malaria/EpidemiologicalData/malaEpi10CasesandDeaths/.

4 Checkley AM, Smith A, Smith V, Blaze M, Bradley D, Chiodini PL, et al. Risk factors for mortality from imported falciparum malaria in the United Kingdom over 20 years: an observational study. *BMJ* 2012;344:bmj.e2116.

5 Ladhani S, Aibara RJ, Riordan FA, Shingadia D. Imported malaria in children: a review of clinical studies. *Lancet Infect Dis* 2007;7:349-57.

6 Green ST, Jary HR, Darton TC. Missed opportunities to diagnose Plasmodium falciparum malaria: results of a regional service evaluation. *J Infect* 2009;58:172-3.

7 Ladhani S, El Bashir H, Patel VS, Shingadia D. Childhood malaria in East London. *Pediatr Infect Dis J* 2003;22:814-9.

8 Dubos F, Dauriac A, El Mansouf L, Courouble C, Aurel M, Martinot A. Imported malaria in children: incidence and risk factors for severity. *Diagn Microbiol Infect Dis* 2010;66:169-74.

9 World Health Organization. Guidelines for the treatment of malaria. 2 edn. WHO, 2010.

10 Centers for Disease Control and Prevention. Domestic refugee health guidelines: malaria. secondary domestic refugee health guidelines: malaria. 2012. www.cdc.gov/immigrantrefugeehealth/guidelines/domestic/malaria-guidelines-domestic.html.

11 Newman RD, Parise ME, Barber AM, Steketee RW. Malaria-related deaths among U.S. travelers, 1963-2001. *Ann Intern Med* 2004;141:547-55.

12 Svenson JE, MacLean JD, Gyorkos TW, Keystone J. Imported malaria. Clinical presentation and examination of symptomatic travelers. *Arch Intern Med* 1995;155:861-8.

13 Batwala V, Magnussen P, Nuwaha F. Are rapid diagnostic tests more accurate in diagnosis of plasmodium falciparum malaria compared to microscopy at rural health centres? *Malar J* 2010;9:349.

14 Lalloo DG, Shingadia D, Pasvol G, Chiodini PL, Whitty CJ, Beeching NJ, et al. UK malaria treatment guidelines. *J Infect* 2007;54:111-21.

15 Abba K, Deeks JJ, Olliaro P, Naing CM, Jackson SM, Takwoingi Y, et al. Rapid diagnostic tests for diagnosing uncomplicated P. falciparum malaria in endemic countries. *Cochrane Database Syst Rev* 2011;(7):CD008122.

16 Rossi I, D'Acremont V, Prod'Hom G, Genton B. Safety of falciparum malaria diagnostic strategy based on rapid diagnostic tests in returning travellers and migrants: a retrospective study. *Malar J* 2012;11:377.

17 D'Acremont V, Landry P, Mueller I, Pecoud A, Genton B. Clinical and laboratory predictors of imported malaria in an outpatient setting: an aid to medical decision making in returning travelers with fever. *Am J Trop Med Hyg* 2002;66:481-6.

18 Bottieau E, Clerinx J, Colebunders R, Van den Enden E, Wouters R, Demey H, et al. Selective ambulatory management of imported falciparum malaria: a 5-year prospective study. *Eur J Clin Microbiol Infect Dis* 2007;26:181-8.

19 Kiang KM, Bryant PA, Shingadia D, Ladhani S, Steer AC, Burgner D. The treatment of imported malaria in children: an update. *Arch Dis Child Educ Pract Ed* 2013;98:7-15.

20 Dondorp A, Nosten F, Stepniewska K, Day N, White N, South East Asian Quinine Artesunate Malaria Trial (SEAQUAMAT) group. Artesunate versus quinine for treatment of severe falciparum malaria: a randomised trial. *Lancet* 2005;366:717-25.

21 Dondorp AM, Fanello CI, Hendriksen ICE, Gomes E, Seni A, Chhaganlal KD, et al. Artesunate versus quinine in the treatment of severe falciparum malaria in African children (AQUAMAT): an open-label, randomised trial. *Lancet* 2010;376:1647-57.
22 British Medical Association, Royal Pharmaceutical Society of Great Britain. British national formulary. London: BMA, RPS, 2013:422, 428. (No 65.)

Human brucellosis

Brodie Ramin, family medicine resident[1],
Paul MacPherson, associate professor[2]

[1]Ottawa Hospital, University of Ottawa, Ottawa, Canada, K1H 8L6

[2]Division of Infectious Diseases, Ottawa Hospital, Ottawa Health Research Institute, University of Ottawa, Canada

Correspondence to: Brodie Ramin bramin@ottawahospital.on.ca

Cite this as: BMJ 2010;341:c4545

DOI: 10.1136/bmj.c4545

www.bmj.com/content/341/bmj.c4545

Brucellosis is the most common bacterial zoonosis, with over 500 000 new cases globally every year.[1] Human brucellosis is transmitted primarily through unpasteurised dairy products derived from infected animals. The disease has also been known as "Malta fever" and "Mediterranean fever."[2] *Brucella* species are small Gram negative coccobacilli that are facultative intracellular pathogens for humans; the most common animal reservoirs for human disease are sheep and goats.[3]

Why is brucellosis missed?

Case reports have shown delays of several months in the diagnosis of brucellosis, increasing the morbidity for affected patients.[3] Brucellosis is missed for two reasons. Firstly, like tuberculosis and syphilis, the disease is a great "imitator" and can present with non-specific features in any organ system.[4] Secondly, brucellosis is rare in western Europe and North America and so is often not considered in the differential diagnosis, even in patients with clear risk factors, and is often mistaken for tuberculosis, malaria, or typhoid fever.[3]

Why does it matter?

Although brucellosis in human beings is rarely fatal, it can be severely debilitating. Furthermore, the disease tends to be chronic and may persist for several years.[5] It is associated with a 5% overall mortality rate, predominantly from endocarditis.[4] Early recognition and treatment can shorten the course of illness and prevent complications.[6] Brucellosis is a notifiable disease in most jurisdictions, including the United Kingdom.

How is it diagnosed?

Brucellosis is usually contracted through consuming unpasteurised dairy products, especially raw milk, soft cheese, butter, and ice cream.[6] Travellers who have consumed unpasteurised dairy products from regions where *Brucella* is endemic are at high risk. The highest annual rates of human brucellosis are found in Middle Eastern countries, the former Soviet republics of central Asia, parts of Latin America, and most Mediterranean countries; additionally, although the disease is believed to be endemic in India, there are no national incidence data.[1]

Brucellosis can also be transmitted through occupational exposure; it is the most commonly reported laboratory associated bacterial infection.[7] Inhalation and direct contact with *Brucella* organisms can also cause infection in abattoir workers, meat packers, and veterinarians.[6]

KEY POINTS

- Brucellosis is the most common bacterial zoonosis, with over 500 000 cases globally every year
- Brucellosis is most often contracted through consuming unpasteurised dairy products, especially raw milk, soft cheese, butter, and ice cream
- The most common features of the disease are fever, malaise, headache, back pain, night sweats, and arthritis; endocarditis is the most common cause of the 5% mortality rate
- The optimal treatment regimen is oral doxycycline with either rifampicin or parenteral streptomycin or gentamicin in the initial period

How common is human brucellosis?

Country	No of annual cases per million population
Syria	1600
Kyrgyzstan	360
Iraq	280
Turkey	260
Tunisia	35
Mexico	29
Greece	21
United States	0.4
United Kingdom	0.3

Data comes from Pappas et al, 2006.[1]

CASE SCENARIO

A 38 year old woman presents to her general practitioner complaining of 10 weeks of fatigue and joint pains. She had returned from Turkey three months before, and while there she had had a one week episode of fevers. When questioned about food consumption abroad, she admits eating local cheese while travelling in rural Turkey. On examination, she has mild hepatomegaly, but there are no other findings. Serology tests confirm human brucellosis.

TREATMENT GUIDELINES FOR BRUCELLOSIS[10]

- Oral regimen: 100 mg doxycycline twice daily plus 600-900 mg of rifampicin once daily for a minimum of six weeks
- Oral/parenteral regimen: 100 mg doxycycline orally twice daily for six weeks and either 15 mg/kg streptomycin intramuscularly daily or gentamicin 5 mg/kg daily parenterally for the first 21 days

Clinical features

After infection the period of incubation lasts two to eight weeks.[6] The most common clinical features are fever (74% of cases) and constitutional symptoms (26%) such as malaise, anorexia, and night sweats.[8] Arthritis (22%) is usually migratory and predominantly affects large joints.[3] Physical findings may be few on examination. Hepatomegaly and splenomegaly are detected in about a third of patients.[9] Lymphadenopathy is seen in about 7% of patients.[6] Malodorous perspiration is almost pathognomonic for brucellosis.[6]

Neurological findings are present in about 6% of cases, ranging from peripheral neuropathies to meningoencephalitis.[4, 8] Respiratory disease, including pleural effusions and pneumonia, can complicate the course of the infection.[4] Endocarditis, typically involving the aortic valve, occurs in less than 2% of cases but remains the principal cause of mortality from brucellosis.[6] In pregnancy, *Brucella* infection leads to increased rates of spontaneous abortion in the first trimester.[3]

Investigations

The definitive test for diagnosis is blood cultures, which have a sensitivity of 20-80%.[4] In the absence of culture facilities, various serological tests are available, such as the rose bengal test and a serum agglutination test.[4] Physicians should consult their local laboratories to determine availability of diagnostic tests. Other investigations should include a complete blood count (to detect leucocytopenia, lymphocytosis, thrombocytopenia, anaemia), liver enzymes (for mild transaminitis), C reactive protein, and erythrocyte sedimentation rate (mildly raised in brucellosis), and cultures of infected organs if indicated (bone marrow, cerebrospinal fluid, joint fluid, ascitic fluid).[8]

How is it managed?

The World Health Organization's guidelines for the treatment of brucellosis were set out in 1986. The 2007 Ioannina recommendations updated the guidelines with the addition of gentamicin as equivalent to streptomycin for the initial period (box).[10] Treatment failure rates are much higher with the oral regimen.[4]

Physicians should educate all patients travelling to regions where *Brucella* is endemic about measures to prevent infection in the first place. Travellers should practise safe eating habits—in particular, they should avoid raw milk and undercooked meat and should avoid "traditional" (unpasteurised) forms of dairy products.[3]

Contributors: BR and PMacP contributed equally to this paper. BR is the guarantor.

Funding: No special funding.

Competing interests: All authors have completed the Unified Competing Interest form and declare that BR and PM have no support for the submitted work; BR and PM have no relationships that might have an interest in the submitted work in the previous three years; their spouses, partners, or children have no financial relationships that may be relevant to the submitted work; and BR, PM have no non-financial interests that may be relevant to the submitted work.

Provenance and peer review: Not commissioned; externally peer reviewed.

Patient consent not required (patient anonymised, dead, or hypothetical).

1 Pappas G, Papdimitriou P, Akritidis N, Christou L, Tsianos EV. The new global map of human brucellosis. *Lancet Infect Dis* 2006;6:91-9

2 Nicoletti P. A short history of brucellosis. *Vet Microbiol* 2002;90:5-9.

3 Memish ZA, Balkhy HH. Brucellosis and international travel. *J Travel Med* 2004;11:49-55.

4 Franco MP, Mulder M, Gilman RH, Smits HL. Human brucellosis. *Lancet Infec Dis* 2007;7:775-86.

5 Vassalos CM, Economou V, Vassalou E, Papadopoulou C. Brucellosis in humans: why is it so elusive? *Rev Med Microbiol* 2009;20:63-73.

6 Pappas G, Akritidis N, Bosilkovski M, Tsianos E. Brucellosis. *N Engl J Med* 2005;352:2325-36.

7 Centers for Disease Control and Prevention. Brucellosis. 2007. www.cdc.gov/ncidod/dbmd/diseaseinfo/Brucellosis_g.htm.

8 Buzgan T, Karahocagil MK, Irmak H, Baran AI, Karsen H, Evirgen O, et al. Clinical manifestations and complications in 1028 cases of brucellosis: a retrospectic evaluation and review of the literature. *Int J Infect Dis* [forthcoming].

9 Andriopulos P, Tsironi M, Deftereos S, Aesspopos A, Assimakopoulos G. Acute brucellosis: presentation, diagnosis, and treatment of 144 cases. *Int J Infect Dis* 2007;11:52-7.

10 Ariza J, Bosilkovski M, Cascio A, Colmenero JD, Corbel MJ, Falagas ME, et al. Perspectives for the treatment of brucellosis in the 21st century: the Ioannina recommendations. *PLoS Medicine* 2007;4:1872-8.

Whooping cough

Anthony Harnden, university lecturer in general practice[1]

[1]Department of Primary Health Care, University of Oxford, Oxford OX3 7LF

Correspondence to: anthony.harnden@dphpc.ox.ac.uk

Cite this as: *BMJ* 2009;338:b1772

DOI: 10.1136/bmj.b1772

www.bmj.com/content/338/bmj.b1772

Whooping cough is a common respiratory infection caused by the bacterium *Bordetella pertussis*. It should be considered as a possible diagnosis in any adolescent or adult with an acute cough of more than two weeks' duration, even if they have been fully immunised.

Why is it missed?

In the post-vaccination era, whooping cough is under-recognised in primary care as the incidence is incorrectly thought to be low. The classic clinical features of whooping cough, such as an inspiratory "whoop" (listen on bmj.com), may be attenuated in older children and adults who have been immunised.[1] Moreover, many doctors may not be aware that there is a simple diagnostic serological test.

Why does this matter?

A persistent cough without explanation can cause distress and anxiety, and the patient may be subject to inappropriate investigations, treatment, and referral.[5] Secondly, early diagnosis and treatment with erythromycin can prevent the patient transmitting their infection within and outside the household.[6] This may be especially important in young infants, who may have severe complications such as respiratory failure and death.[7] Thirdly, notification of all cases of whooping cough by primary care clinicians and enhanced surveillance of laboratory proved cases would give a better estimate of the efficacy of the vaccine and of the burden of disease in the community.

How is it diagnosed?

Clinical features

Acute cough persisting for more than two weeks, without the characteristic inspiratory whoop, may be the only clinical symptom of whooping cough. Initial symptoms, lasting for up to two weeks, mimic a simple upper respiratory tract infection. This is the most infectious period. Paroxysmal episodes of coughing may continue for up to six weeks but can recur with further respiratory infections. In China whooping cough is referred to as the one hundred day cough. In all age groups, irrespective of immunisation status, the cough lasts an average of three months.

Investigations

Bordetella pertussis is a difficult organism to culture without a correctly collected pernasal swab or nasopharyngeal aspirate; neither of these samples is easy to collect in primary care. The sensitivity of culture falls from 15-45% to 0% during the first three weeks of the cough, and sensitivity may be further reduced by antibiotic treatment, previous immunisation, and transport of the specimen.[8]

KEY POINTS

- Consider a diagnosis of whooping cough in any patient with an acute persistent cough of more than two weeks' duration
- A single raised IgG titre to pertussis toxin is 99% specific for diagnosis and is the recommended test in primary care
- Oral erythromycin taken within 21 days of the onset of the cough may prevent transmission
- Notification of all cases of whooping cough by primary care clinicians, and enhanced surveillance of laboratory proved cases, would give a better estimate of vaccine efficacy and the burden of disease in the community

CASE SCENARIO

A 17 year old girl presents with a three week history of cough. The cough keeps her awake at night and she has bouts of coughing that disturb her classmates. She is fully immunised. Her general practitioner requests serology for anti-pertussis toxin IgG antibodies, which are found to be raised, indicating a recent infection with *Bordetella pertussis*.

HOW COMMON IS IT?

Whooping cough is a statutory notifiable disease in the United Kingdom, but notifications remain low. Yet epidemiological evidence indicates that whooping cough remains an endemic disease in adolescents and adults.[2] International case series of adolescents and adults with cough lasting for two weeks or more have reported that about 20% of individuals have evidence of recent whooping cough.[3] Serological surveys have shown that whooping cough occurs repeatedly throughout adult life, and it has been estimated people have up to three episodes in a lifetime, despite immunisation.[4]

Serology is the recommended diagnostic blood test in primary care and is routinely used in many countries: a single raised titre of antipertussis toxin IgG has a sensitivity of 76% and a specificity of 99% for the diagnosis of whooping cough across all age groups.[9] More recently, assays of antipertussis toxin IgG levels in oral fluid have been validated; they are quick and simple to use in primary care and have recently been made available in the UK.[10]

How is it managed?

Whooping cough should be notified. Treatment may not affect outcome for the patient, but erythromycin within 21 days of onset of symptoms reduces the period of infectivity and may prevent transmission to household members.[6] A seven day course is sufficient. Prophylaxis with erythromycin should be offered to everyone in households with a vulnerable infant who may be unimmunised or partly immunised.[6] In infants the illness may be severe and require prompt referral to secondary care.

I thank Doug Jenkinson for permission to use an audio clip from his website and for his work in promoting the clinical recognition of whooping cough in primary care.

Funding: No external funding.

Competing interests: AH has an ongoing interest in pertussis research and is conducting studies involving the use of oral fluid antibody testing.

Provenance and peer review: Not commissioned; externally peer reviewed.

1 Harnden A, Grant C, Harrison T, Perera R, Brueggemann AB, Mayon-White R, et al. Whooping cough in school age children with persistent cough: a prospective cohort study in primary care *BMJ* 2006;333:174-7.
2 Wright SW, Edwards KM, Decker MD, Zeldin MH. Pertussis infection in adults with persistent cough. *JAMA* 1995;273:1044-6.
3 Cagney M, MacIntyre CR, McIntyre P, Torvaldsen S, Melot V. Cough symptoms in children aged 5-14 years in Sydney, Australia: non-specific cough or unrecognized pertussis? *Respirology* 2005;10:359-64.
4 De Melker HE, Versteegh FG, Schellekens JF, Teunis PF, Kretzshmar M. The incidence of Bordetella pertussis infections estimated in the population from a combination of serological surveys. *J Infect* 2006;53:106-13.
5 Levenson R. A patient's journey: whooping cough. *BMJ* 2007;334:532-3.
6 Dodhia H, Crowcroft NS, Bramley JC, Miller E. UK guidelines for use of erythromycin chemoprophylaxis in persons exposed to pertussis. *J Public Health Med* 2002;24:200-6.
7 Crowcroft NS, Andrews N, Rooney C, Brisson M, Miller E. Deaths from pertussis are underestimated in England. *Arch Dis Child* 2002;86:336-8.
8 Crowcroft NS, Peabody RG. Recent developments in pertussis *Lancet* 2006;367:1926-36.
9 De Melker HE, Versteegh FG, Conyn-van Spaendonck, Elvers LH, berbers GA, van der Zee A, et al. Specificity and sensitivity of high levels of immunoglobulin G antibodies against pertussis toxin in a single serum sample for diagnosis of infection with Bordetella pertussis. *J Clin Microbiol* 2000;38(2):800-6.
10 Litt DJ, Samuel D, Duncan J, Harnden A, George RC, Harrison TG. Detection of anti-pertussis toxin IgG in oral fluids for use in diagnosis and surveillance of Bordetella pertussis infection in children and young adults. *J Med Microbiol* 2006;55:1223-8.

Syphilitic condylomata lata mimicking anogenital warts

F G Bruins, dermatologist-venereologist[1],
F J A van Deudekom, resident in internal medicine[2],
H J C de Vries, dermatologist-venereologist[3 4 5]

[1]Clinic for Dermatology, DermaPark, Uden, Netherlands

[2]Department of Internal Medicine, Kennemergasthuis, Haarlem, Netherlands

[3]Department of Dermatology, Academic Medical Centre, University of Amsterdam, 1100 DD Amsterdam, Netherlands

[4]STI Outpatient Clinic, Public Health Service Amsterdam, Amsterdam, Netherlands

[5]Centre for Infection and Immunity Amsterdam (CINIMA), Academic Medical Center, University of Amsterdam, Amsterdam, Netherlands

Correspondence to: H J C de Vries h.j.devries@amc.nl

Cite this as: *BMJ* 2015;350:h1259

DOI: 10.1136/bmj.h1259

http://www.bmj.com/content/350/bmj.h1259

A 41 year old man who has sex with men visited our dermatology outpatient clinic with a three month history of non-painful anal papules. He reported protected anal contact with multiple (anonymous) male partners.

Physical examination showed perianal flesh coloured papules with a verrucous surface (fig 1). One papule showed partial ulceration. Our differential diagnosis was between human papillomavirus (HPV) associated genital warts and condylomata lata, a cutaneous manifestation seen in secondary syphilis. On histopathological examination of a lesional biopsy, immunostaining for *Treponema pallidum* showed a dense plasma-cellular infiltrate and numerous spirochetes. An HPV specific nucleic acid amplification test did not detect viral DNA in the biopsy. The diagnosis was confirmed by serological testing with a *T pallidum* specific enzyme immunoassay and the Venereal Disease Research Laboratory (VDRL) test; HIV-1 and HIV-2 serology were both negative. He was given intramuscular injections of 2.4×10^6 IU benzathine benzylpenicillin, and the lesions had disappeared completely at a follow-up visit.

What are condylomata lata?

These are one of the cutaneous signs of secondary syphilis. They reside in skin folds, such as those seen in the inguinal, perianal, and perivaginal regions and appear as flat papules with a moist, cauliflower-like or velvety surface. Moreover, they contain numerous spirochetes and are highly infectious (fig 2A).[1] They can mimic anogenital warts (condylomata acuminata), which are associated with HPV infection, and are characterised by verrucous or papilliform, pink or skin coloured papules (fig 2B).[2]

How common are they?

Between 2012 and 2013 the overall incidence of infectious syphilis in England increased by 9%—3249 cases were reported.[3] In genitourinary medicine clinics, syphilis is mainly seen in men who have sex with men, with 81% (2393/2970) of cases in men being in this group.

THE BOTTOM LINE

- Condylomata lata are a cutaneous manifestation of secondary syphilis and can be misdiagnosed as genital warts
- Prompt diagnosis and treatment with intramuscular benzathine benzylpenicillin are needed to prevent serious neurological complications (such as syphilitic meningitis and cerebrovascular disease), cardiac complications (such as aortic valve destruction), and ongoing transmission
- Initial diagnostic tests includes an anti-treponemal serological assay and an anticardiolipin test
- Once condylomata lata are suspected, refer promptly to a specialist centre such as a sexual health clinic or to a (dermato-)venereologist for further investigations (including sexually transmitted infection screen), treatment, contact tracing, and follow-up

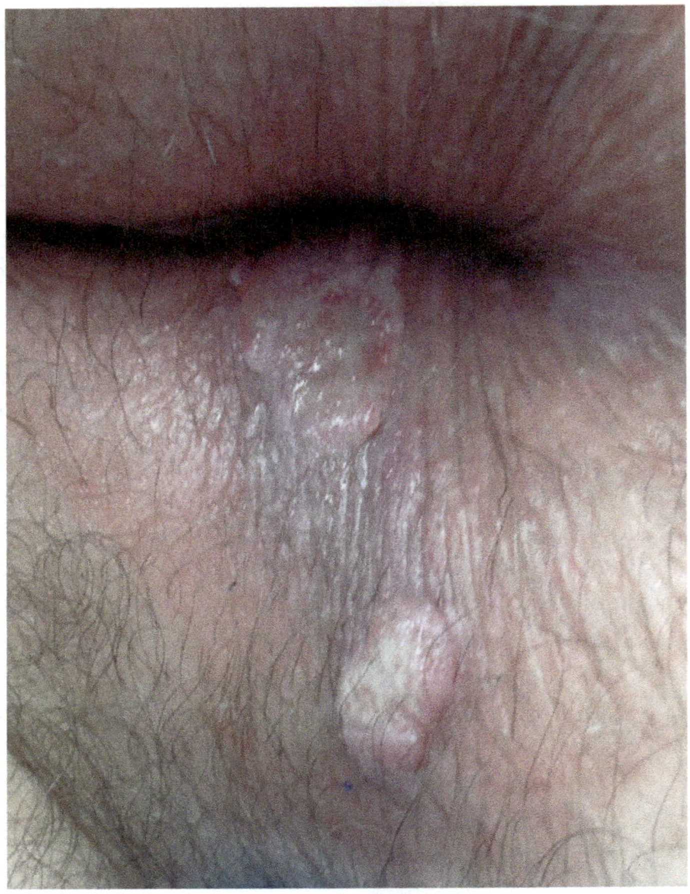

Fig 1 Condylomata lata in a man with secondary stage syphilis characterised by verrucous hyperkeratotic perianal papules. The condylomata latum on top shows partial ulceration

Why are they missed?

Because of the painless nature of condylomata lata patients can easily miss these lesions, especially if they are located at an internal site such as the anus, vagina, or mouth. Moreover, they can easily be mistaken by doctors for another dermatological condition such as anogenital warts (fig 2B), bowenoid papulosis, HPV induced anal intraepithelial neoplasia, or skin tags.[4]

Why does this matter?

Misdiagnosis delays adequate treatment and results in ongoing transmission to sex partners. Syphilis is treated completely differently from genital warts. If untreated, syphilis can have irreversible consequences, including neurosyphilis (such as syphilitic meningitis and cerebrovascular disease) and cardiovascular disease (such as aortic valve destruction).

How are they diagnosed?

Clinical

Condylomata lata are characteristic of secondary syphilis. By contrast, the primary stage of syphilis is characterised by a small painless, indurated ulcer, typically with rolled edges, which is accompanied by regional lymphadenopathy. Secondary syphilis can present with a variety of symptoms, most often a maculopapular rash, but also alopecia, leucoplakic or erythematous lesions on oral mucous membranes, and perianal or perivaginal condylomata lata.

Investigations

A clinical suspicion of syphilis is initially confirmed by serology, using an anti-treponemal serological assay (for example, the *T pallidum* enzyme immunoassay, which is usually reported as positive or negative or as a semi quantitative index; or the *T pallidum* haemagglutination assay (TPHA)) and an anticardiolipin test (such as the VDRL test, reported

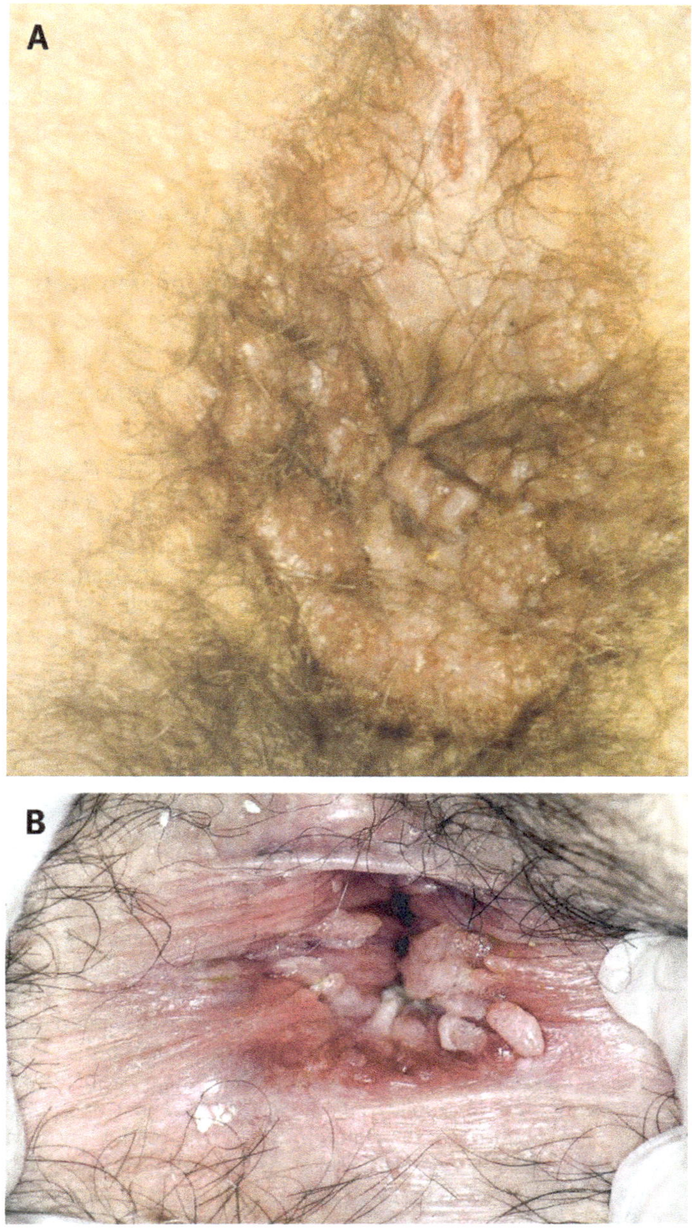

Fig 2 (A) Perianal condylomata lata with a typical verrucous aspect. (B) Perianal and intra-anal genital warts characterised by verrucous papules

as titre). In primary syphilis, serological tests can be falsely negative in the window phase, so serology may need to be re-evaluated after several weeks; the TPHA and VDRL tests have 70.4% and 74.9% sensitivity, respectively. In secondary syphilis serological testing is highly sensitive—98.6% and 97.4% for TPHA and VDRL tests, respectively[5]; VDRL also usually shows a high titre (>1:16).

In specialist clinics, dark field microscopy may be used to diagnose ulcerative primary stage lesions and condylomata lata, by visualising *T pallidum* in lesional exudate. This is a cheap and quick diagnostic method but requires a specialised microscope and expertise.

To differentiate syphilitic condylomata from HPV induced manifestations, such as genital warts or bowenoid papulosis, a biopsy is needed for histopathological examination. A dense plasma cell infiltrate and numerous spirochetes visualised by immunostaining confirm condylomata lata. Numerous nucleic acid amplification tests to detect *T pallidum* have been developed in house but are not available routinely. These tests are highly specific and sensitive in the diagnosis of primary syphilis, irrespective of the serological window phase.[6]

How are they managed?

It is advisable to refer patients suspected of having syphilis to a specialised setting, such as a sexual health or infectious diseases clinic, or to a (dermato-)venereologist, where additional investigations and treatment are readily available and contact tracing and follow-up can be offered.

The primary, secondary, and early latent stages of syphilis can easily be treated with a single intramuscular 2.4×10^6 IU dose of benzathine benzylpenicillin. Patients diagnosed as having syphilis should always undergo tests for other sexually transmitted diseases, including HIV and hepatitis B serology, and nucleic acid amplification testing of urine, vaginal, anorectal or pharyngeal swabs (depending on the patient's sexual practices) for chlamydia and gonorrhoea. Furthermore, partner notification is needed to prevent transmission, although this may be a problem when sexual contacts are anonymous.[7] Men who have sex with men who often have new or casual partners are advised to be screened for sexually transmitted infections and HIV every three months.[3]

Contributors: FGB, FJvD, and HJdV all contributed to the acquisition, analysis, conception, design, drafting, and revision of the work and its intellectual content; gave their final approval of the version to be published; and agreed to be accountable for all aspects of the work in ensuring that questions related to the accuracy or integrity of any part of the work are appropriately investigated and resolved. HJdV is guarantor.

Competing interests: We have read and understood BMJ policy on declaration of interests and declare the following interests: none.

Provenance and peer review: Not commissioned; externally peer reviewed.

Patient consent not required (patient anonymised, dead, or hypothetical).

1 De Vries HJ. Skin as an indicator for sexually transmitted infections. *Clin Dermatol* 2014;32:196-208.
2 Edwards L, Lynch PJ, eds. *Genital dermatology atlas.* 2nd ed. Wolters Kluwer Lippincott Williams & Wilkins, 2011:205.
3 Public Health England. Sexually transmitted infections and chlamydia screening in England 2013. Health protection report. Vol 8, No 24. 2014. www.gov.uk/government/uploads/system/uploads/attachment_data/file/345181/Volume_8_number_24_hpr2414_AA_stis.pdf.
4 Gearhart PA, Randall TC, Buckley RM, et al. Human papillomavirus differential diagnoses. http://emedicine.medscape.com/article/219110-differential.
5 Anderson J, Mindel A, Tovey SJ, et al. Primary and secondary syphilis, 20 years' experience. 3: diagnosis, treatment, and follow up. *Genitourin Med* 1989;65:239-43.
6 Heymans R, van der Helm JJ, de Vries HJ, et al. Clinical value of Treponema pallidum real-time PCR for diagnosis of syphilis. *J Clin Microbiol* 2010;48:497-502.
7 Kohl KS, Farley TA, Ewell J, et al. Usefulness of partner notification for syphilis control. *Sex Transm Dis* 1999;26:201-7.

Herpes simplex virus encephalitis

Raymond Egdell, patient's father[1],
Darren Egdell, patient[2],
Tom Solomon, professor of neurological science[3], director[4]

[1]Worsley, UK

[2]Leigh, UK

[3]Walton Centre NHS Foundation Trust, Liverpool L9 7LJ, UK

[4]Institute of Infection and Global Health, University of Liverpool, Liverpool L69 7BE

Correspondence to: T Solomon tsolomon@liverpool.ac.uk

Cite this as: *BMJ* 2012;344:e3630

DOI: 10.1136/bmj.e3630

www.bmj.com/content/344/bmj.e3630

This is one of a series of occasional articles by patients about their experiences that offer lessons to doctors. The *BMJ* welcomes contributions to the series. Please contact Peter Lapsley (plapsley@bmj.com) for guidance.

Darren Egdell developed herpes simplex virus encephalitis 10 years ago, aged 31. He and his father, Raymond, look back at the initial illness and describe his remarkable progress.

Raymond—the patient's father

When Darren first became ill, the doctor diagnosed flu; and all the symptoms pointed to flu. It was only two days later, when he woke one morning mumbling and incomprehensible, that his mum and I realised there was more to it than flu. We phoned an ambulance straight away.

A young doctor rushed into the accident and emergency department, and I feared the worst. He said it was either meningitis, a growth on the brain, or encephalitis. I didn't want to think about meningitis or a growth on the brain, and I'd never heard of encephalitis before, so I told him that if I could choose, I would have that. But he told me that was the last one I should pick, because it was the worst. Fortunately it didn't take long for the doctors to reach a diagnosis and start the treatment with aciclovir. They saved Darren's life. Without a diagnosis and treatment at that point, they would not have been able to do anything for him.

He was in hospital for about six weeks. We were there all day, every day. But it was hard. For a couple of weeks we didn't know whether he would survive or not; but even when he did, nobody told us what sort of person we would be taking home from the hospital. When he came round, he didn't know who we were. And bizarrely, he couldn't speak any English at first, only French. He had done French at university and spoken it fluently. But his mum and I don't speak French so it was impossible to converse with him. We had to have a translator to talk to our own son. He had a terrible temper and argumentative side to begin with; and he swore, which he had never done before. It wasn't Darren that we had brought home; it was a different person. He had been allowed home for a weekend, and didn't know where he was. At the end of the weekend, when it was time to go back to the hospital, he very politely thanked me and his mum for having him. It was heartbreaking at the time.

Each day in hospital the specialist would come and see him, and ask him to name things in English. Darren could describe how a fountain pen worked in minute detail, and what it was for; but he couldn't actually tell you what it was called. The doctor would ask him who the prime minister was. Hour after hour I would drum it into him "Tony Blair, Tony Blair." But he still couldn't remember. He had to relearn everything. He didn't know simple words such as knife, fork, or spoon. First we played easy word games with him then moved on to Scrabble. He played again and again and again, until he could beat us both, as before. But to this day he still can't remember the names of animals.

I had been so proud of how bright Darren was before his illness. He was a member of MENSA and had his French degree and a high powered job. Then to see it all disappear in a matter of a few days was unbelievable—to know his brain is never going to be the same again, that he's never going to be able to use it the way he did. All gone. That's very hard to accept. But he has done so well, worked so hard, to get this far. I am proud of him for that. Over the years he has got rid of the temper and got back to being the lovely person

A DOCTOR'S PERSPECTIVE

Herpes simplex virus encephalitis is the most commonly diagnosed viral encephalitis in the United Kingdom, with an annual incidence estimated at 2-4 per million. Although in the 1980s the mortality improved with the introduction of aciclovir, the morbidity remains high, especially when treatment is started late. Recent work by our group, and others, looking at where the delays occur and why, has resulted in the development of new national encephalitis guidelines (see "Useful resources" box), which should encourage better management.

In Darren's case there were no delays in treatment. He was admitted to hospital on the day he developed altered consciousness; in retrospect, the apparently disgusting smell of food was probably an olfactory hallucination, which may be an early clue to herpes encephalitis. In hospital the constellation of a febrile illness and abnormal behaviour was quickly recognised as an indicator of possible brain infection; the lumbar puncture was consistent with viral disease, and aciclovir was started, all within a few hours of admission. However, Darren's outcome shows that despite rapid treatment, the effect of herpes simplex virus on the brain can still be catastrophic, both for the patient and the family. The importance of the Encephalitis Society in helping Darren and his family to cope with the illness is also very apparent.

Herpes simplex virus type 1 is transmitted through droplets and is thought to enter the central nervous system via the olfactory nerve, which sends branches to the temporal lobes, hence the characteristic damage to this part of the brain in herpes encephalitis. The medial temporal lobe, especially the hippocampus, is important in laying down new memories (anterograde memory); this explains why anterograde memory is so often affected in herpes encephalitis. In Darren's case, in addition to anterograde amnesia, there is memory loss for events before the illness—retrograde amnesia. His knowledge of facts, semantic memory, is also affected, with a striking inability to recall the names of common objects. Perhaps most extraordinary of all, though, is that despite his difficulties with English, Darren's French language skills were relatively preserved. Whereas verbal memory is strongly left lateralised in the medial temporal lobe, learning of foreign language is thought to reside in the right hemisphere; and clearly in Darren's case this has made an enormous difference to the sequelae of his disease.

But beyond the fascinating insights it gives us into how the brain works, this case highlights the need for further research on disease mechanisms in encephalitis, and the role of anti-inflammatory treatments as adjuncts to antiviral drugs.

Tom Solomon, professor of neurological science

he was. When I compare him with others we meet through the Encephalitis Society, I realise how much he has improved.

The Encephalitis Society has been a real lifesaver for us. We go for trips, and it is clear some people have been affected even more than Darren. Four of them went to McDonald's; they put their order in, but by the time the food came, only two minutes later, no one could remember what they'd asked for. He goes on holiday with one friend from the society. They went to France in the car. Darren can remember the names of places, but she can't. She can remember the routes, but he can't. So between them they get there.

Darren

I don't remember much about being ill. I can remember going to my girlfriend's house for something to eat, but it was weird; the food smelt disgusting and made me sick. I went to bed on the Saturday night feeling tired, and with a headache. On the Sunday when I woke my speech wasn't making sense. I thought I was talking normally, but I wasn't. I couldn't understand why everyone was looking at me strangely.

When I was recovering, the doctors would always ask me the same questions. They wanted to know who the prime minister was. Once, I gave them a perfect description: a woman, blond, pearl necklace, always wears blue, and carries a handbag. And the doctors laughed because apparently I'd given a perfect description of the prime minister, but the wrong one. She had been replaced 10 years earlier. They would show me pictures, but I

USEFUL RESOURCES

- Encephalitis Society (www.encephalitis.info/)—Offers support for those affected by encephalitis, raises awareness, and promotes research
- Solomon T, Michael BD, Smith PE, Sanderson F, Davies NWS, Hart IJ, et al. Management of suspected viral encephalitis in adults—Association of British Neurologists and British Infection Association National Guidelines. *J Infection* 2012;64:347-73
- Kneen R, Michael BD, Menson E, Mehta B, Easton A, Hemingway C, et al. Management of suspected viral encephalitis in children—Association of British Neurologists and British Paediatric Allergy, Immunology and Infection Group National Guidelines. *J Infect* 2012;64:449-77
- www.braininfectionsuk.org/—A portfolio of research studies aimed at improving the outcome of encephalitis and other central nervous system infections of major importance in the UK
- Liverpool Neurological Infections Diseases Course (www.liv.ac.uk/neuroidcourse/)—An annual course for clinicians of all specialties who want to update their knowledge and improve their skills

couldn't name the objects. Some I still struggle with—for example, the thing you get near the North Pole; it's made of ice; like a circle; it has a door on it; you can go inside; all the blocks of ice are put together; it has to be cold there, otherwise the ice melts. I can tell you all about it, but can never remember what it is called.

I watch French DVDs with English subtitles, to help me learn the English words again; then I watch the film again in English, and see if I can understand it. I read books in French, especially kids' books. I like the Roald Dahl and Harry Potter books. Unlike adult books, children's keep repeating the same words, again and again. This helps you remember them. But I struggle with names. For example, I can remember Harry Potter, and Ron Weasley; but I can never remember the name of the girl. Even though I know it starts with H and has eight letters.

I have little ways of trying to remember names. My next door neighbour, for example, is a bit shorter than me; so instead of Darren, his name is shorter—Dan. Sometimes if I can't remember an English word, I'll think of the French, and that helps me get there. It can be embarrassing in a supermarket. I am looking for something and can't find it; then by the time I've got the attention of the staff, I've forgotten the name of the thing I am looking for.

Moving into my current house, with three floors, was difficult at first. I'd be in the kitchen and need something from the top floor. By the time I got there I'd have forgotten what I wanted. That happens to everyone. But I'd then get back down to the kitchen, realise what I needed, and go up and down, three or four times, until in the end, I learnt to write a Post-it note, and stick it on the back of my hand, so I know what I am looking for. I dictate into a Dictaphone to keep a diary of what needs doing, and I leave notes everywhere. And I have to keep everything organised in exactly the right place, otherwise I can never find things.

The Encephalitis Society has a retreat every two years in Wales, which is the most brilliant thing. It is for people who have had encephalitis, so it is not embarrassing. The first time I went there I met a man who said "my memory is not that bad; I know your name is Darren and you are from the north west." But at dinner time, he kept asking for more and more soup, because he couldn't remember he had just had some! It is weird; everyone has different memory problems. One man went to the toilet, and got lost on his way back; he ended up knocking on the window. I was in hysterics. It was so great to meet others who have similar problems.

Competing interests: All authors declare no support from any organisation for the submitted work; no financial relationships with any organisations that might have an interest in the submitted work in the previous three years, no other relationships or activities that could appear to have influenced the submitted work.

Provenance and peer review: Not commissioned; not externally peer reviewed.

PVL positive *Staphylococcus aureus* skin infections

A Fogo, dermatology registrar[1],
N Kemp, general practitioner[2],
R Morris-Jones, consultant dermatologist[1]

[1]Dermatology Department, King's College Hospital, London SE5 9RS, UK

[2]Elm Lodge Surgery, London SE24 9HJ

Correspondence to: A Fogo abigailfogo@nhs.net

Cite this as: *BMJ* 2011;343:d5343

DOI: 10.1136/bmj.d5343

www.bmj.com/content/343/bmj.d5343

Patients presenting with recurrent skin abscesses may be infected with the rapidly emerging and highly pathogenic strains of *Staphylococcus aureus* that carry the virulence factor Panton-Valentine leukocidin (PVL). PVL positive *S aureus* can be acquired in the community and lead to recurrent and potentially serious infections of the skin and necrotising pneumonia.

Why is PVL positive *S aureus* skin infection missed?

Although PVL positive *S aureus* skin infections can be suspected on clinical grounds (severity and extent of lesions, similar lesions in close contacts, frequency of relapse, and poor response to normally effective chemotherapy), it can only be confirmed by taking swabs from lesional skin, any pus, and carrier sites. The clinician must then ask the microbiology laboratory to test any *S aureus* isolates for the presence of PVL genes. PVL gene detection is not routinely tested in the UK and therefore must be specifically asked for on the request form when sending swabs. Antibiotic sensitivities alone cannot be relied on to discriminate between PVL positive and PVL negative strains of *S aureus*.

Why does it matter?

In patients with many boils or abscesses, the delayed identification of PVL positive *S aureus* can lead to serious morbidity over many months. PVL positive *S aureus* is associated with higher morbidity and mortality, and is also highly transmissible, when compared with PVL negative *S aureus*.[5] Patients may have time off work, make frequent appointments at their general practice for wound management, and take many courses of antibiotics that are clinically ineffective. The highly transmissible nature of PVL positive *S aureus* means that onward transmission is more likely with prolonged infections owing to delayed diagnosis or inadequate treatment. Rarely, PVL positive *S aureus* infections can become invasive, leading to necrotising haemorrhagic pneumonia (mortality approaching 75%[6]), necrotising fasciitis, and purpura fulminans. A quarter of patients with PVL necrotising pneumonia give a history of previous skin lesions (boils) themselves or in close family contacts.[5] From a public health perspective, early recognition and treatment of PVL positive *S aureus* infections in the UK should help to prevent the rapid rise in PVL community infections that has been seen in the United States.

KEY POINTS

- The prevalence of PVL positive *Staphylococcus aureus* in the community is rapidly increasing
- Suspect PVL positive *S aureus* infection when patients present with recurrent boils, particularly when there is a history of similar lesions in household members or close contacts
- Send microbiology samples specifically requesting PVL gene detection, as well as microscopy, culture, and sensitivity

How is PVL positive *S aureus* skin infection diagnosed?

Clinical

Patients are usually healthy young adults.[5] Guidance from the Centers for Disease Control and Prevention refers to the "five Cs" of risk factors for PVL related infection: contaminated items; close contact; crowding; cleanliness; and cuts and compromised skin integrity.[7] In North America, settings identified as higher risk for transmission include households, close contact sports, gyms, and prisons.[5]

Patients present to their general practitioner with a history of recurrent boils or abscesses (from two to over 15 such skin lesions) over weeks or months, and other family members or contacts may be similarly affected. Our 39 year old patient (figure) presented with recurrent, deep, painful abscesses over 12 months.

Investigations

In patients with recurrent boils, necrotising skin, or soft tissue infections, when there is someone else in the household with such symptoms or if the patient is in a closed community, take a microbiology swab from infected skin and nares. Request microscopy, culture, and sensitivities, and also ask the laboratory to test for the presence of PVL positive *S aureus*.

How is PVL positive *S aureus* skin infection managed?

Most cases of PVL positive *S aureus* in the UK are currently sensitive to flucloxacillin, erythromycin, and clindamycin. The current guidelines from the Health Protection Agency recommend a seven day course of oral flucloxacillin or clindamycin for meticillin sensitive strains. They advise treating PVL positive meticillin resistant *S aureus* isolates with rifampicin and one other agent (clindamycin, doxycycline, sodium fusidate, or trimethoprim). In our experience in secondary care, patients that we saw with PVL positive meticillin sensitive *S aureus* infections had already failed treatment with flucloxacillin in the community. The reasons for this are not clear; however, laboratory data relating to the management of necrotising pneumonia caused by PVL positive *S aureus* suggest that flucloxacillin may, in fact, increase PVL production.[3] [9] Suboptimal tissue concentrations of flucloxacillin within necrotic lesions are also thought to be partly responsible, whereas clindamycin

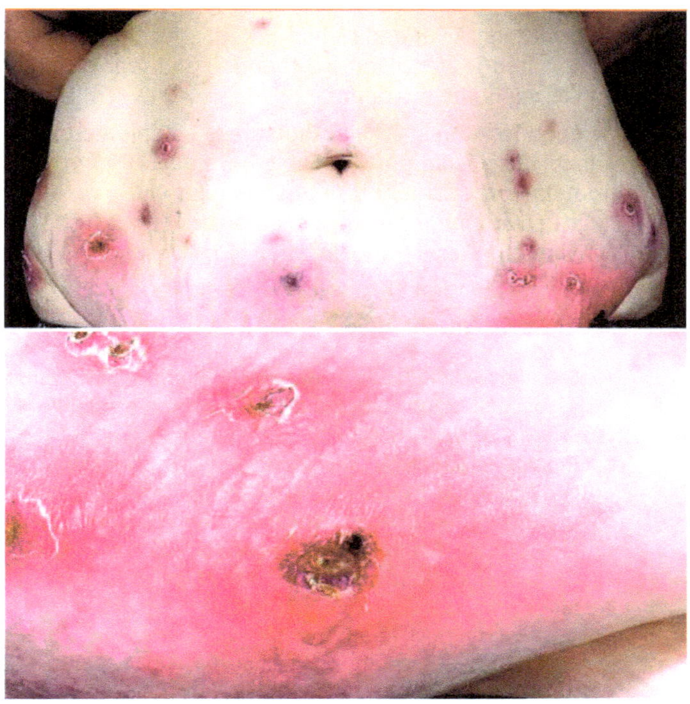

Fig 1 Top: Necrotising abscesses typical of PVL positive *S aureus* infection. Bottom: Cutaneous abscess with purulent discharge, central ulceration, and severe soft tissue inflammation

CASE SCENARIO

A 39 year old woman presented with recurrent deep painful abscesses (figure) and was one of 30 similar patients referred to our dermatology unit over the past 12 months. She was otherwise well with no intercurrent illness. Routine skin swabs taken by her general practitioner grew meticillin sensitive *S aureus*, but the abscesses did not resolve after several weeks of oral flucloxacillin. Further swabs were therefore taken and the *S aureus* isolate was sent to the national staphylococcal reference unit for typing. This confirmed PVL positive *S aureus*, which is not easily eradicated from skin infections with conventional courses of flucloxacillin or erythromycin. The patient subsequently required a four week course of rifampicin and clindamycin, plus five days of chlorhexidine wash and nasal mupirocin, to clear the lesions completely. No relapse was seen six months later.

HOW COMMON IS PVL POSITIVE *S AUREUS* SKIN INFECTION?

- Recent (2010) data from the United Kingdom found that 20% of *S aureus* isolates from skin or soft tissue infections contained PVL positive *S aureus*,[1] and although the sample may have been biased towards the more severe skin or soft tissue infections, this prevalence is far higher than the 2% recorded in 2005.[2 3]
- Worldwide literature reports similar figures—for example, in one study, 30% of 100 consecutive *S aureus* isolates from patients with skin or soft tissue infections that were analysed in a German university hospital laboratory were PVL positive.[4]
- Currently, PVL associated with meticillin sensitive *S aureus* is less common in the UK than in the United States.[5] The prevalence in the UK of PVL positive meticillin resistant *S aureus* (MRSA) isolates from skin infections is currently estimated to be about 0.8%.[1]
- Of the 30 cases of PVL positive *S aureus* causing recurrent boils seen in our unit over the past 12 months, three (10%) were PVL positive MRSA isolates.

and rifampicin have good soft tissue penetration and work synergistically. Furthermore, to interrupt transmission of PVL positive *S aureus*, the HPA guidelines suggest that all patients plus their close contacts are treated with topical decolonisation for five days (chlorhexidine 4% wash to the body daily and mupirocin ointment applied three times daily to the anterior nares).

Contributors: AF and RM-J had the idea for the article and did the literature search. All authors contributed to the planning, conduct, and reporting of the article. All authors together wrote the article. AF is the guarantor.

Competing interests: All authors have completed the ICMJE uniform disclosure form at www.icmje.org/coi_disclosure.pdf (available on request from the corresponding author) and declare: no support from any organisation for the submitted work; no financial relationships with any organisation that might have an interest in the submitted work in the previous three years; no other relationships or activities that could appear to have influenced the submitted work.

Provenance and peer review: Not commissioned; externally peer reviewed.

Patient consent obtained.

1 Shallcross LJ, Williams K, Hopkins S, Aldridge RW, Johnson AM, Hayward AC. Panton-Valentine leukocidin associated staphylococcal disease: a cross-sectional study at a London hospital, England. *Clin Microbiol Infect* 2010;16:1644-8.

2 Holmes A, Ganner M, McGuane S, Pitt TL, Cookson BD, Kearns AM. *Staphylococcus aureus* isolates carrying Panton-Valentine leucocidin genes in England and Wales: frequency, characterization, and association with clinical disease. *J Clin Microbiol* 2005;43:2384-90.

3 Ellington MJ, Ganner M, Smith IM, Perry C, Cookson BD, Kearns AM. Panton-Valentine leucocidin-related disease in England and Wales. *Clin Microbiol Infect* 2010;16:86-8.

4 Monecke S, Slickers P, Ellington MJ, Kearns AM, R Ehricht. High diversity of Panton-Valentine leukocidin-positive, methicillin-susceptible isolates of Staphylococcus aureus and implications for the evolution of community-associated methicillin-resistant S. aureus. *Clin Microbiol Infect* 2007;13:1157-64.

5 Health Protection Agency. Guidance on the diagnosis and management of PVL-associated Staphylococcus aureus infections (PVL-SA) in the UK. 2008. www.hpa.org.uk/webc/HPAwebfile/HPAweb_C/1218699411960.

6 McGrath B, Rutledge F, Broadfield E. Necrotising pneumonia, Staphylococcus aureus and Panton-Valentine-Leukocidin. *JICS* 2008;9:170-2.

7 Hawkes M, Barton M, Conly J, Nicolle L, Barry C, Ford-Jones EL. Community-associated MRSA: superbug at our doorstep. *CMAJ* 2007;176(1):54-6.

8 Stevens DL, Ma Y, McIndoo E, Wallace RJ, Bryant A. Impact of antibiotics on expression of virulence-associated exotoxin genes in methicillin-sensitive and methicillin-resistant Staphylococcus aureus. *J Infect Dis* 2007;195:202-11.

9 Dumitrescu O, Boisset S, Badiou C, Bes M, Benito Y, Reverdy M-E, et al. Effect of antibiotics on staphylococcus aureus producing Panton-Valentine leukocidin. *Antimicrob Agents Chemother* 2007;51:1515-9.

BPP UNIVERSITY SCHOOL OF HEALTH BMJ

Appendicitis

Sian R R Lewis, locum general practitioner[1],
Peter J Mahony, general practitioner[2],
John Simpson, associate professor in gastrointestinal surgery[3]

[1]Nottingham, UK

[2]Belvoir Health Group, The Surgery, Nottingham, UK

[3]Department of General Surgery, University Hospital/Queens Medical Centre, Nottingham NG7 2UH, UK

Correspondence to: J Simpson j.simpson@nottingham.ac.uk

Cite this as: *BMJ* 2011;343:d5976

DOI: 10.1136/bmj.d5976

www.bmj.com/content/343/bmj.d5976

Acute appendicitis is the most common abdominal condition requiring emergency surgery. It results from inflammation of the vermiform appendix, which is a tubular structure attached to the base of the caecum.

Why is appendicitis missed?

The classical presentation of appendicitis appears in only approximately 50% of patients.[4] Appendicitis can affect all age groups, and presentation may be influenced by the patient's age and the anatomical position of the appendix. An accurate history may not be possible from the very young or from older people presenting with confusion.

Pregnancy seems to protect against appendicitis,[5] but it is the most common non-obstetric emergency requiring surgery in pregnancy. Presentations in pregnant women may be atypical (due to anatomical displacement of the appendix by the gravid uterus) or mistaken for the onset of labour; tenderness may be located anywhere on the right side of the abdomen or may be minimal if the inflamed appendix is displaced posterolaterally.

The diagnostic accuracy of general practitioners in relation to appendicitis is high (92% of paediatric cases correctly diagnosed) and the non-specificity of symptoms and signs is the predominant reason for a delay in diagnosis.[6]

Why does this matter?

Appendicitis is a progressive inflammatory process, and the incidence of perforated cases rises with the duration of symptoms. Therefore, prompt diagnosis and treatment are essential for reducing the increased risk associated with advanced inflammation. After the first 36 hours following the onset of symptoms the average rate of perforation is between 16% and 36%, and the risk of perforation is 5% for every subsequent 12 hour period.[7] Perforation rates are higher in elderly people and young children,[8] possibly because of a delay in diagnosis.[9] However, actual perforation rates are difficult to calculate accurately due to the frequency of undiagnosed cases of resolving appendicitis.[10]

How is appendicitis diagnosed?

Clinical features

Diagnosis of acute appendicitis relies on a thorough history and examination, and the presence or absence of any particular individual symptom or sign cannot be relied upon to diagnose or exclude appendicitis.

In the assessment of a patient with suspected appendicitis, studies have demonstrated that pain migration (positive likelihood ratio 2.06) and evidence of peritoneal irritation (localised direct or indirect tenderness (1.29-2.47), rigidity (2.96), guarding (2.48), rebound

KEY POINTS

- Appendicitis is a predominantly clinical diagnosis, and no single individual symptom or sign can be relied upon to diagnose or exclude it
- A history of fever or pain migration and evidence of peritoneal irritation have been found to be the most useful clinical features in making the diagnosis
- A raised CRP and white cell count can support the diagnosis
- The classical presentation can be influenced by the age of the patient and anatomical position of the appendix

(1.99), and percussion tenderness (2.86) are the most useful clinical findings associated with a positive diagnosis.[11]

Abdominal pain is the primary presenting complaint of patients with acute appendicitis. However, the sequence of vague abdominal pain followed by vomiting with migration of the pain to the right iliac fossa first described by Murphy may be present only in around 50% of patients.[4] Typically, the patient describes a periumbilical or epigastric pain that intensifies during the first 24 hours, becoming constant and sharp, and migrates to the right iliac fossa. Loss of appetite is often a predominant feature, and constipation and nausea are frequently present. Profuse vomiting is rarely a major feature in simple appendicitis. The patient can be flushed, with a dry tongue and associated fetor oris. The presence of pyrexia (up to 38°C) with tachycardia is common. Abdominal examination reveals localised tenderness and muscular rigidity after localisation of the pain to the right iliac fossa. The site of maximal tenderness is often said to be over McBurney's point, which lies two thirds of the way along a line drawn from the umbilicus to the anterior superior iliac spine. Rebound tenderness is present but the test should be used with caution as it can be distressing for the patient. Movement frequently exacerbates the pain, and asking patients to cough will often localise the pain to the right iliac fossa. Demonstration of Rovsing's sign (palpation of the left iliac fossa causes pain in the right iliac fossa due to peritoneal irritation) may also aid in the diagnosis of appendicitis. In atypical cases, clinical assessment of the right groin and hip is important, particularly in paediatric patients, to rule out pathology in this region.

Scoring systems

Scoring systems have been developed to aid the diagnosis of appendicitis. They aim to estimate the probability of the condition in an individual patient compared with a large number of similar patients from which the system was developed. The best known of the several systems developed is the Alvarado score,[12] although more recently the appendicitis inflammatory response (AIR) score correctly classified a higher proportion of patients into low probability and high probability groups. The scores use history and examination findings along with inflammatory markers to achieve a summed numerical score. In a study of 545 patients with suspected appendicitis the receiver operating characteristic area for the AIR score was 0.93 compared to 0.88 for the Alvarado score (P=0.0007).[13]

Anatomical considerations in the presentation of acute appendicitis

- Retrocaecal/retrocolic (20%)[14] – Right loin pain is often present, with tenderness on examination. Muscular rigidity and tenderness to deep palpation are often absent because of protection from the overlying caecum. The psoas muscle may be irritated in this position, leading to hip flexion and exacerbation of the pain on hip extension (psoas stretch sign)
- Subcaecal and pelvic (51%)[14] – Suprapubic pain and urinary frequency may predominate. Diarrhoea and tenesmus may be present as a result of irritation of the rectum. Abdominal tenderness may be lacking, but rectal or vaginal tenderness may be present on the right. Microscopic haematuria and leukocytes may be present on urinalysis
- Pre-ileal and post-ileal (25%)[14] – Diarrhoea may result from irritation of the distal ileum. A presumptive diagnosis of gastroenteritis may delay a diagnosis of appendicitis[8]

Investigations

There is no specific laboratory test for appendicitis although simple blood tests may support the diagnosis as the majority of patients with appendicitis will have a neutrophil predominant leukocytosis. Combining C-reactive protein and white cell count can provide a likelihood ratio for appendicitis of up to 23.32 depending on values taken.[11] In contrast, when all inflammatory markers are normal, appendicitis is unlikely.[11]

To assess for obstetric related conditions, pregnancy testing is mandatory in women of child bearing age.

CASE SCENARIO

A 50 year old man presented with a 24 hour history of generalised abdominal pain that had become localised in the right loin. He had no urinary symptoms but was feverish (37.8°C). His urine was positive for blood and protein, and a provisional diagnosis of renal colic was made. He was referred to hospital, where computed tomography of the kidneys, ureters, and bladder did not demonstrate any evidence of urinary calculi but did confirm the presence of an inflamed retrocaecal appendix. He underwent an open appendicectomy and made an uneventful recovery.

HOW COMMON IS APPENDICITIS?

- Appendicitis is the most common abdominal emergency and accounts for more than 40 000 hospital admissions in England every year (approximately 1 per 1500 population)[1]
- Appendicitis is most common between the ages of 10 and 20 years, but no age group is exempt
- There is a male to female ratio of 1.4:1; overall lifetime risk is 8.6% for males and 6.7% for females in the United States[2]
- Since the 1940s the incidence of hospital admission for acute appendicitis has been falling, but the reason for this decline is not clear[3]

Urinalysis may be abnormal in almost half of patients with acute appendicitis because of inflammation adjacent to the right sided urinary tract and bladder.[15]

Appendicitis is predominantly a clinical diagnosis that can be supported by simple blood tests—specialist tests aren't usually required. However, the most frequently used radiological investigations are ultrasonography (sensitivity and specificity of 86% and 81%) and computed tomography (94% and 95%),[16] although the latter should be used with caution to minimise radiation exposure.

How is appendicitis managed?

Appropriate resuscitation followed by expedient appendicectomy either by the open or laparoscopic approach is the treatment of choice. All patients should receive broad spectrum perioperative antibiotics as this decreases the incidence of postoperative wound infections and abscess formation.[17]

Contributors: SRRL and JS wrote the first draft. PJM made important revisions. JS is guarantor.

Competing interests: All authors have completed the ICMJE uniform disclosure form at www.icmje.org/coi_disclosure.pdf (available on request from the corresponding author) and declare: no support from any organisation for the submitted work; no financial relationships with any organisations that might have an interest in the submitted work in the previous three years, no other relationships or activities that could appear to have influenced the submitted work. JS declares that MA Healthcare paid travel expenses and accommodation fees for speaking at an educational event on the subject of acute appendicitis in September 2010.

Provenance and peer review: Commissioned; externally peer reviewed.

Patient consent not required (patient anonymised, dead, or hypothetical).

1 Hospital Episode Statistics. Primary diagnosis: summary. www.hesonline.nhs.uk/Ease/servlet/ContentServer?siteID=1937&categoryID=202.
2 Addiss DG, Shaffer N, Fowler BS, Tauxe RV. The epidemiology of appendicitis and appendectomy in the United States. *Am J Epidemiol* 1990;132:910-25.
3 Kang JY, Hoare J, Majeed A, Williamson RC, Maxwell JD. Decline in admission rates for acute appendicitis in England. *Br J Surg* 2003;90:1586-92.
4 Murphy JB. Two thousand operations for appendicitis, with deductions from his personal experience. *Am J Med Sci* 1904;128:187-211.
5 Andersson RE, Lambe M. Incidence of appendicitis during pregnancy. *Int J Epidemiol* 2001;30:1281-5.
6 Wilson D, Sinclair S, McCallion WA, Potts SR. Acute appendicitis in young children in the Belfast urban area: 1985-1992. *Ulster Med J* 1994;63:3-7.
7 Bickell NA, Aufses AH Jr, Rojas M, Bodian C. How time affects the risk of rupture in appendicitis. *J Am Coll Surg* 2006;202:401-6.
8 Cappendijk VC, Hazebroek FW. The impact of diagnostic delay on the course of acute appendicitis. *Arch Dis Child* 2000;83:64-6.

9 Hale DA, Molloy M, Pearl RH, Schutt DC, Jaques DP. Appendectomy: a contemporary appraisal. *Ann Surg* 1997;225:252-61.
10 Andersson RE. The natural history and traditional management of appendicitis revisited: spontaneous resolution and predominance of prehospital perforations imply that a correct diagnosis is more important than an early diagnosis. *World J Surg* 2007;31:86-92.
11 Andersson RE. Meta-analysis of the clinical and laboratory diagnosis of appendicitis. *Br J Surg* 2004;91:28-37.
12 Alvarado A. A practical score for the early diagnosis of acute appendicitis. *Ann Emerg Med* 1986;15:557-64.
13 Andersson M, Andersson RE.The appendicitis inflammatory response score: a tool for the diagnosis of acute appendicitis that outperforms the Alvarado score. *World J Surg* 2008;32:1843-9.
14 Ahmed I, Asgeirsson KS, Beckingham IJ, Lobo DN. The position of the vermiform appendix at laparoscopy. *Surg Radiol Anat* 2007;29:165-8.
15 Puskar D, Bedalov G, Fridrih S, Vuckovic I, Banek T, Pasini J. Urinalysis, ultrasound analysis, and renal dynamic scintigraphy in acute appendicitis. *Urology* 1995;45:108-12.
16 Terasawa T, Blackmore CC, Bent S, Kohlwes RJ. Systematic review: computed tomography and ultrasonography to detect acute appendicitis in adults and adolescents. *Ann Intern Med* 2004;141:537-46.
17 Andersen BR, Kallehave FL, Andersen HK. Antibiotics versus placebo for prevention of postoperative infection after appendicectomy. *Cochrane Database Syst Rev* 2005;3:CD001439.

BPP UNIVERSITY SCHOOL OF HEALTH BMJ

Bronchiectasis

Nick H T ten Hacken, associate professor, pulmonary department, Thys van der Molen, professor, general practitioner department

University Medical Center Groningen, University of Groningen, 9713 GZ Groningen, Netherlands

Correspondence to: N H T ten Hacken n.h.t.ten.hacken@long.umcg.nl

Cite this as: *BMJ* 2010;341:c2766

DOI: 10.1136/bmj.c2766

www.bmj.com/content/341/bmj.c2766

Bronchiectasis is mostly an acquired bronchopulmonary disorder with abnormal thickening of the bronchial wall and dilation of central and medium sized bronchi, due to a vicious circle of transmural infection and inflammation with mediator release. Though many underlying conditions may induce or contribute to the development of bronchiectasis (table), it is idiopathic in about 50% of adults[1] and 25% of children.[2]

How common is it?

The prevalence of bronchiectasis varies with time period and geography, due to differences in antibiotic prescription, availability of vaccinations, and prevalence of associated disorders. Additionally, the doctor's alertness for bronchiectasis and the availability of sensitive diagnostic tools may affect reported prevalence. In the United States the prevalence of non-cystic fibrosis bronchiectasis among adults between 1999 and 2001 was estimated to be 51 per 100 000 population.[3] The prevalence was higher among women than men (71 *v* 32 per 100 000) and increased markedly with age (4 per 100 000 for people aged 18-34 years *v* 272 per 100 000 for those aged 75 or over). In Australia the prevalence among Aboriginal children aged under 15 years was reported to be as high as 1470 per 100 000.[4]

In the United Kingdom, a full time, single handed practice of 2500 patients will have one or two patients with bronchiectasis, compared with 75 with asthma and 50 with chronic obstructive pulmonary disease.

Why is it missed?

Symptoms of bronchiectasis (such as chronic cough and sputum production) may be mild, particularly at the beginning. These symptoms may resemble asthma, chronic obstructive pulmonary disease, rhinosinus diseases, tracheobronchial infection, and gastroesophageal reflux, which are much more common than bronchiectasis in an average UK general practice. In an Australian cohort study, 40% of patients with bronchiectasis who developed chronic productive cough in adulthood also smoked.[5] This may mislead the doctor to a diagnosis of chronic bronchitis induced by smoking. Basal crackles may suggest heart failure. Spirometry may show coexisting airway obstruction, leading to a misdiagnosis of chronic obstructive pulmonary disease instead of bronchiectasis. Chest x rays sometimes do not show mild bronchiectasis.

KEY POINTS

- Bronchiectasis may be easily missed because its clinical features may overlap with more common conditions, such as asthma, chronic obstructive pulmonary disease, rhinosinus disease, gastroesophageal reflux, and common upper and lower airway infections
- General practitioners in the UK have one or two patients, on average, with bronchiectasis in their practice
- Diagnosis is based on daily production of mucopurulent phlegm and chest imaging that shows dilated and thickened airways; high resolution computed tomography of the lung is the optimum diagnostic procedure
- The diagnosis of bronchiectasis should lead to investigation and treatment of possible causes and associated conditions
- Treat acute exacerbations promptly with short courses (less than four weeks) of antibiotics

Causes of and conditions associated with bronchiectasis[1]

Cause	No (%) (n=150)
Idiopathic	80 (53)
Infection	44 (29)
Immune defect	12 (8)
Congenital	1 (<1)
Condition	
Allergic bronchopulmonary aspergillosis	11 (7)
Aspiration	6 (4)
Young's syndrome	5 (3)
Cystic fibrosis	4 (3)
Rheumatoid arthritis	4 (3)
Ciliary dysfunction	3 (2)
Ulcerative colitis	2 (<1)
Panbronchiolitis	1 (<1)

In this case series no patients were found with $\alpha 1$ antitrypsin deficiency, but in a case series of 74 patients deficient in $\alpha 1$ antitrypsin, 70 were found to have bronchiectatic changes.[17]

Why does it matter?

Patients with newly diagnosed bronchiectasis were found to have a poorer prognosis than those with asthma (matched for age and sex), but a better prognosis than those with chronic obstructive pulmonary disease.[6] Over a follow-up period of 8.8 years, 25% of 372 Finnish patients with bronchiectasis died (mean age at the start of the follow-up was 56 years). In a Turkish cohort study in 98 patients with bronchiectasis, vaccination, scheduled visits to the doctor, and high body mass index seemed to improve survival.[7]

No controlled intervention studies have been done on the effect of an early diagnosis, a higher alertness of the general practitioner, or an active screening programme. Nevertheless, evidence based guidelines of the American College of Chest Physicians say that once bronchiectasis is discovered, looking for an underlying cause is important, as the results of diagnostic evaluation "may lead to treatment that may slow down or halt the progression of the disease."[8] The diseases that are described as underlying causes are among others listed in table 1.

How is it diagnosed?

Clinical features

Cough is present in 90% of the patients, and 76% produce sputum daily.[9] Haemoptysis occurs in 51% of patients and tends to be recurrent. The usual abnormalities on chest examination are crackles (70%) and wheezes (34%).

Investigations

Requesting sputum cultures in patients with frequent respiratory infections may help to identify unusual infections that increase the suspicion of bronchiectasis, as the case scenario shows. Chest x rays may show linear markings, crowding, cystic spaces, and honeycombing.[10] In a small study the sensitivity for chest x rays to detect bronchiectasis was found to be 88%, with a specificity of 74%,[11] but other studies indicate that these figures will be less positive in mild bronchiectasis.

A normal chest x ray does not exclude bronchiectasis definitively. So, if there is a high clinical suspicion for bronchiectasis, a high resolution computed tomography scan of the chest should be considered. This scan has replaced contrast bronchography as optimal for diagnosis of bronchiectasis. Major features are airway dilation, lack of tapering (figure), thickening of the bronchial wall, mucopurulent plugs or debris, and cysts.[12] The sensitivity of the scan is 82-97% and the specificity 99-100%.[13]

Specific tests to identify underlying causes or contributing conditions depend on the clinical setting and the patient's history and age. Tests might include a white blood cell

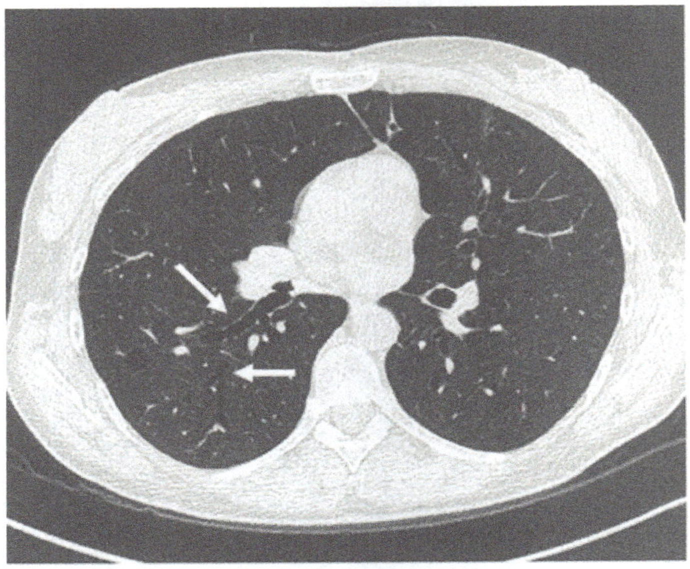

High resolution computed tomography scan of chest of a young non-smoking woman with mild bronchiectasis. White arrows indicate airway dilation and lack of tapering

CASE SCENARIO

A 29 year old, non-smoking kindergarten teacher with mild asthma often visited her general practitioner with recurrent respiratory tract infections, which they both attributed to daily contact with her students. After seven courses of oral antibiotics in one year, the doctor requested sputum cultures. These showed *Pseudomonas aeruginosa*. Given this unusual result and her recurrent infections, he referred her to a lung physician, and high resolution computed tomography of her lung showed mild bronchiectasis, which was later found to be due to $\alpha 1$ antitrypsin deficiency.

count and differentiation, IgG, IgG subclasses, IgM, IgA, total IgE, $\alpha 1$ antitrypsin levels, rheumatoid factor, and aspergillus serology.

How is it managed?

The evidence base for management is contentious, but expert consensus advocates advising patients who smoke to quit. Treat acute exacerbations with short courses (<4 weeks) of antibiotics targeted to likely organisms such as *Pseudomonas aeruginosa, Haemophilus influenza,* or *Mycobacterium avium-intracellulare*; or on basis of the results of sputum culture. Consider prolonged use of antibiotics (>4 weeks)[14]; although the criteria for doing so are not well established, we believe this might be beneficial in patients who often relapse (more than six times per year) or show progressive decline of lung function. The effectiveness of continuous mucolytics, anti-inflammatory agents, and bronchodilators is not clear but can be considered on individual basis.[15] Physical therapy techniques that improve bronchial clearance of mucus are widely used, yet there is little evidence to support or refute them.[16]

Contributors: NHTH and TvdM both did the research and revision; NHTH wrote the first version. NHTH is guarantor.

Funding: No additional funding.

Competing interests: All authors have completed the Unified Competing Interest form at www.icmje.org/coi_disclosure.pdf (available on request from the corresponding author) and declare (1) no support from any company for the submitted work; (2) no relationships with any companies that might have an interest in the submitted work in the previous 3 years; (3) their spouses, partners, or children have no financial relationships that may be relevant to the submitted work; and (4) no non-financial interests that may be relevant to the submitted work.

Provenance and peer review: Not commissioned; externally peer reviewed.

Patient consent not required (patient anonymised, dead, or hypothetical).

1 Pasteur MC, Helliwell SM, Houghton SJ, Webb SC, Foweraker JE, Coulden RA, et al. An investigation into causative factors in patients with bronchiectasis. *Am J Respir Crit Care Med* 2000;162:1277-84.
2 Li AM, Sonnappa S, Lex C, Wong E, Zacharasiewicz A, Bush A, et al. Non-CF bronchiectasis: does knowing the aetiology lead to changes in management? *Eur Respir J* 2005;26:8-14.
3 Weycker D, Edelsberg J, Oster J, Tino G. Prevalence and economic burden of bronchiectasis. *Clin Pulmon Med* 2005;12:205-9.
4 Chang AB, Grimwood K, Mulholland EK, Torzillo PJ. Bronchiectasis in indigenous children in remote Australian communities. *Med J Aust* 2002;177:200-4.
5 King PT, Holdsworth SR, Farmer M, Freezer N, Villanueva E, Holmes PW. Phenotypes of adult bronchiectasis: onset of productive cough in childhood and adulthood. *COPD* 2009;6:130-6.
6 Keistinen T, Saynajakangas O, Tuuponen T, Kivela SL. Bronchiectasis: an orphan disease with a poorly-understood prognosis. *Eur Respir J* 1997;10:2784-7.
7 Onen ZP, Gulbay BE, Sen E, Yildiz OA, Saryal S, Acican T, et al. Analysis of the factors related to mortality in patients with bronchiectasis. *Respir Med* 2007;101:1390-7.
8 Rosen MJ. Chronic cough due to bronchiectasis: ACCP evidence-based clinical practice guidelines. *Chest* 2006;129(suppl):122-31S.
9 Nicotra MB, Rivera M, Dale AM, Shepherd R, Carter R. Clinical, pathophysiologic, and microbiologic characterization of bronchiectasis in an aging cohort. *Chest* 1995;108:955-61.
10 Gudbjerg CE. Roentgenologic diagnosis of bronchiectasis; an analysis of 112 cases. *Acta Radiol* 1955;43:210-26.
11 Van der Bruggen-Bogaarts BA, van der Bruggen HM, van Waes PF, Lammers JW. Screening for bronchiectasis: a comparative study between chest radiography and high-resolution CT. *Chest* 1996;109:608-11.
12 Barker AF. Clinical manifestations and diagnosis of bronchiectasis. UpToDate for Patients. 2008. www.uptodate.com/patients/content/topic.do?topicKey=~MMzSzjTX2Y4
13 Smith IE, Flower CD. Review article: imaging in bronchiectasis. *Br J Radiol* 1996;69:589-93.
14 Evans DJ, Bara AI, Greenstone M. Prolonged antibiotics for purulent bronchiectasis in children and adults. *Cochrane Database Syst Rev* 2007;(2):CD001392.
15 Ten Hacken N, Kerstjens H, Postma D. Bronchiectasis. *Clin Evid (Online)* 2008. http://clinicalevidence.bmj.com/ceweb/conditions/rdc/1507/1507.jsp.
16 Jones AP, Rowe BH. Bronchopulmonary hygiene physical therapy for chronic obstructive pulmonary disease and bronchiectasis. *Cochrane Database Syst Rev* 2000;(2):CD000045.
17 Parr DG, Guest PG, Reynolds JH, Dowson LJ, Stockley RA. Prevalence and impact of bronchiectasis in alpha1-antitrypsin deficiency. *Am J Respir Crit Care Med* 2007;176:1215-21.

Pelvic inflammatory disease

Emily C Bartlett, foundation year 2 doctor in genitourinary medicine[1],
Wendy B Levison, general practitioner[2],
Pat E Munday, retired consultant genitourinary physician[3]

[1]King's College Hospital, Denmark Hill, London SE5 9RS, UK

[2]Callowland Surgery, Watford, Hertfordshire, UK

[3]West Hertfordshire Hospitals NHS Trust, Watford General Hospital, Watford, Hertfordshire, UK

Correspondence to: E C Bartlett Emily.Bartlett@doctors.org.uk

Cite this as: *BMJ* 2013;346:f3189

DOI: 10.1136/bmj.f3189

www.bmj.com/content/346/bmj.f3189

A 22 year old woman in a new sexual relationship presented to her general practitioner with slightly painful intermenstrual bleeding for 10 days. She had pelvic tenderness but no cervical excitation on bimanual examination. The doctor suspected that the bleeding was a side effect of the oral contraceptive pill, started three months earlier. However, as he was unable to rule out pelvic inflammatory disease (PID), endocervical swab samples were taken to test for the sexually transmitted infections caused by *Neisseria gonorrhoeae* and *Chlamydia trachomatis*, and broad spectrum antibiotics prescribed, after which the symptoms resolved. The swab sample confirmed the presence of *C trachomatis*.

What is PID?

PID is due to infection of the upper female genital tract resulting in a wide range of pelvic pathology, from mild endometritis to pelvic peritonitis. Causative organisms are either sexually transmitted (such as *C trachomatis*, *N gonorrhoeae*, *Mycoplasma genitalium*) or endogenous vaginal organisms (for example, *Bacteroides* species) that ascend into the pelvic area from the lower genital tract through the cervix.

Why is PID missed?

PID may present with classic symptoms and signs or with mild and subtle symptoms that may be easy to miss, according to a review of the evidence in national guidelines written by the British Association for Sexual Health and HIV.[2]

The best recent data on easily missed PID come from a retrospective audit in a walk-in centre for sexual health. This showed significantly different rates for the diagnosis of PID among 23 doctors, compared with similar rates for genital warts (a control condition). Although overdiagnosis of PID could not be excluded, the authors postulated that if high diagnosing doctors were overdiagnosing PID, then some women would not display the epidemiological and clinical features of the condition. Instead, the women with a diagnosis by both high and low diagnosing doctors had a similar epidemiological and clinical profile, suggesting underdiagnosis of PID by low diagnosing doctors. It is possible that some doctors may have been looking for severe symptoms, thus having too high a threshold for diagnosis.[3]

Why does this matter?

The sequelae of PID include ectopic pregnancy, infertility, and chronic pelvic pain, and the economic costs of treating these are substantial.[4] The best outcome data on sequelae of PID come from a longitudinal cohort study concerning 2500 women, summarised by Weström et al.[5] A retrospective reanalysis of these data showed that delaying antibiotic treatment for

KEY POINTS

- Consider a diagnosis of PID in young women with any combination of bilateral lower abdominal pain, abnormal vaginal or cervical discharge, abnormal vaginal bleeding, deep dyspareunia, fever, adnexal tenderness, and cervical motion tenderness
- A history of a new sexual partner, change of contraceptive from barrier contraception, or previous PID may be crucial in aiding the diagnosis
- If PID is suspected, treat empirically with a 14 day course of antibiotics to cover *Chlamydia trachomatis, Neisseria gonorrhoeae*, and anaerobes, to achieve clinical and microbiological resolution
- Subsequent infertility may be prevented with early antibiotic treatment

more than three days after the onset of symptoms was associated with a nearly threefold greater risk of post-PID infertility or ectopic pregnancy than in those who sought care promptly (absolute risk 20% *v* 8.3%).[6] A retrospective cohort study in the United States similarly showed that women who had symptoms for two or more days before treatment were more likely to experience infertility than those with symptoms for two or fewer days before treatment (absolute risk 14% *v* 54%).[7] In a third study with a different patient population, the adverse outcomes were less strongly correlated with time to treatment.[8]

How is PID diagnosed?

Clinical

Although not 100% sensitive, laparoscopy is the ideal investigation to diagnosis PID.[9] As this procedure is not available or appropriate in primary care, a clinical diagnosis must be made based on symptoms and signs and the exclusion of competing diagnoses.

PID is most common in women aged 20-29.[1] Historically, the diagnosis of PID has been based on the findings of abdominal tenderness with or without adnexal or cervical excitation tenderness on bimanual examination, with supporting results from investigations confirming an infective or inflammatory process. In one large study of women admitted to hospital with a clinical diagnosis of PID, the sensitivity of abdominal tenderness, cervical motion tenderness, and adnexal tenderness compared with diagnostic laparoscopy was 61.2%, 79.9%, and 90.3% respectively.[10] In a logistic model, the presence of these three signs together was found to be 82.1% sensitive but only 28.6% specific. Other symptoms and signs include nausea or vomiting (sensitivity 27.6%, specificity 69.0%), vaginal discharge (73.1%, 35.7%), vaginal bleeding (16.4%, 73.8%), urinary symptoms (21.6%, 83.3%), proctitis (7.5%, 95.2%), fever (29.9%, 69.0%), and an adnexal mass (90.3%, 21.4%).[9]

Similar studies have confirmed that these symptoms and signs are neither sensitive nor specific when compared with laparoscopy.[11 12] Therefore no combination of symptoms and signs has been adopted in UK national guidelines as the minimal criteria for diagnosis, and a high index of suspicion for PID is recommended.[13]

In practice a thorough history screening for symptoms and a sexual history should be taken. A change of partner or lack of condom use may be important, as sexually transmitted organisms are common causal agents. A history of recent obstetric events (such as vaginal delivery or miscarriage) or gynaecological procedures (such as the insertion of an intrauterine device or termination of pregnancy) is relevant, as disturbance to the cervix may introduce infection to the upper genital tract. Assessment should include an abdominal and vaginal bimanual examination and visualisation of the cervix.

Where the history and examination findings are compatible with a diagnosis of PID, the patient should be treated presumptively.

Investigations

As the diagnosis of PID is made clinically, investigations to confirm an infective or inflammatory process are required to lend support to it. Given the importance of early antibiotic treatment to prevent sequelae, positive results should not be a prerequisite to justify antibiotic treatment.[13]

Endocervical swabs for *C trachomatis* and *N gonorrhoeae*, using nucleic acid amplification tests where available, are recommended in all patients with suspected PID.[2 14] A positive result shows the presence of one of these organisms in the lower genital tract, supporting the diagnosis of PID. However, as these organisms were detected in less than 12% of 22 000 cases of PID seen in genitourinary medicine clinics in England in 2011, a negative swab result does not exclude a diagnosis of PID.[15]

Ultrasound scans are helpful in excluding other diagnostic possibilities, but studies showing both high sensitivity and specificity for PID are lacking.[16]

HOW COMMON IS PID?

- Because of the difficulties in diagnosis, the exact prevalence of PID is not known
- Recent data suggest that the rate of definite PID diagnosis in primary care is about 280/100 000 person years[1]
- This may underestimate the true incidence, as many cases are relatively asymptomatic
- PID is most common in women aged 20-29[1]

An increased erythrocyte sedimentation rate (>15 mm/hr) supports a clinical diagnosis. It is a sensitive (81%) but non-specific (33%) predictor of PID.[17]

Ectopic pregnancy, which is a major differential diagnosis, should be excluded by a pregnancy test.

How is PID managed?

Mild or moderate disease can be safely managed in the outpatient setting, whereas clinically severe disease requires hospital admission for parenteral antibiotics.[2 13] In the outpatient setting, oral antibiotics should be prescribed to cover *C trachomatis, N gonorrhoeae*, and anaerobes.[2 13]

A 14 day course of antibiotics (ceftriaxone, doxycycline, and metronidazole) is recommended, as the optimum treatment duration is unknown, and few data exist to support a shorter course.[18 19] Although some doctors may be concerned about prescribing unnecessary antibiotics, treatment is recommended because the consequences of missing the diagnosis are profound. In those who fail to respond to treatment, laparoscopy is essential to confirm the diagnosis or to make an alternative diagnosis. Once PID has been diagnosed all current sexual partners should be screened and offered empirical treatment, and recent partners (from the previous six months) should be screened for sexually transmitted infections.[2 13]

We thank J Ross for his helpful comments.

Contributors: ECB had the original idea for the paper and wrote the first draft. PEM and WBL revised the manuscript and contributed to the final draft. All authors approved the final version to be published. PEM is the guarantor.

Competing interests: All authors have completed the ICMJE uniform disclosure form at www.icmje.org/coi_disclosure.pdf (available on request from the corresponding author) and declare: no support from any organisation for the submitted work; no financial relationships with any organisations that might have an interest in the submitted work in the previous three years, no other relationships or activities that could appear to have influenced the submitted work.

Provenance and peer review: Not commissioned; externally peer reviewed.

Patient consent not required (patient anonymised, dead, or hypothetical).

1 French CE, Hughes G, Nicholson A, Yung M, Ross JD, Williams T, et al. Estimation of the rate of pelvic inflammatory disease diagnoses: trends in England, 2000-2008. *Sex Transm Dis* 2011;38:158-62.
2 British Association for Sexual Health and HIV. UK national guideline for the management of pelvic inflammatory disease. 2011. www.bashh.org/documents/3572.
3 Doxanakis A, Hayes RD, Chen MY, Gurrin LC, Hocking J, Bradshaw CS, et al. Missing pelvic inflammatory disease? Substantial differences in the rate at which doctors diagnose PID. *Sex Transm Inf* 2008;84:518-23.
4 Yeh JM, Hook EW 3rd, Goldie SJ. A refined estimate of the average lifetime cost of pelvic inflammatory disease. *Sex Transm Dis* 2003;30:369-78.
5 Weström L, Joesoef R, Reynolds G, Hagdu A, Thompson SE. Pelvic inflammatory disease and infertility. *Sex Transm Dis* 1992;19:185-92.
6 Hillis SD, Joesoef R, Marchbanks PA, Wasserheit JN, Cates W Jr, Weström L. Delayed care of pelvic inflammatory disease as a risk factor for impaired fertility. *Am J Obstet Gynecol* 1993;168:1503-9.
7 Safrin S, Schachter J, Dahrouge D, Sweet RL. Long-term sequelae of acute pelvic inflammatory disease: a retrospective cohort study. *Am J Obstet Gynecol* 1992;166:1300-5.
8 Taylor BD, Ness RB, Darville T, Haggerty CL. Microbial correlates of delayed care for pelvic inflammatory disease. *Sex Transm Dis* 2011;38:434-8.
9 Sellors J, Mahony J, Goldsmith C, Rath D, Mander R, Hunter B, et al. The accuracy of clinical findings and laparoscopy in pelvic inflammatory disease. *Am J Obstet Gynecol* 1991;164(Pt 1):113-20.

10 Morcos R, Frost N, Hnat M, Petrunak A, Caldito G. Laparoscopic versus clinical diagnosis of acute pelvic inflammatory disease. *J Reprod Med* 1993;38:53-6.
11 Bevan CD, Johal BJ, Mumtaz G, Ridgway GL, Siddle NC. Clinical, laparoscopic and microbiological findings in acute salpingitis: report on a United Kingdom cohort. *Br J Obstet Gynaecol* 1995;102:407-14.
12 Gaitán H, Angel E, Diaz R, Parada A, Sanchez L, Vargas C. Accuracy of five different diagnostic techniques in mild-moderate pelvic inflammatory disease. *Infect Dis Obstet Gynecol* 2002;10:171-80.
13 Royal College of Obstetricians and Gynaecologists. Management of acute pelvic inflammatory disease. Guideline 32. 2008. www.rcog.org.uk/files/rcog-corp/uploaded-files/T32PelvicInflamatoryDisease2008MinorRevision.pdf.
14 British Association for Sexual Health and HIV. UK National guideline on gonorrhoea testing. 2012. www.bashh.org/documents/4490.
15 Health Protection Agency Statistics. 2013. www.hpa.org.uk/webc/HPAwebFile/HPAweb_C/1215589015024.
16 Munday P. Pelvic inflammatory disease—an evidence-based approach to diagnosis. *J Infect* 2000;40:31-40.
17 Simms I, Warburton F, Weström L. Diagnosis of pelvic inflammatory disease: time for a rethink. *Sex Transm Infect* 2003;79:491-4.
18 Ross J. Pelvic inflammatory disease. *Clin Evid* 2008;3:1606.
19 Walker C, Wiesenfeld H. Antibiotic therapy for acute pelvic inflammatory disease: the 2006 centres for disease control and prevention sexually transmitted diseases treatment guidelines. *Clin Infect Dis* 2007;44:S111-22.

Endometriosis

Samuel Engemise, clinical research fellow in obstetrics and gynaecology[1], Cerys Gordon, general practitioner[2], Justin C Konje, professor of obstetrics and gynaecology[1]

[1]Reproductive Sciences Section, Department of Cancer Studies and Molecular Medicine, University Hospitals of Leicester NHS Trust and University of Leicester, Leicester LE2 7LX

[2]South Wigston Health Centre, Wigston LE18 4SE

Correspondence to: J C Konje jck4@le.ac.uk

Cite this as: *BMJ* 2010;340:c2168

DOI: 10.1136/bmj.c2168

www.bmj.com/content/340/bmj.c2168

Endometriosis is the presence of functional endometrial glands and stroma at various extrauterine sites in women, predominantly those of reproductive age, from all ethnic and social groups. It is a common, benign, oestrogen dependent, chronic gynaecological disorder and a common cause of chronic pelvic pain in women presenting in primary care. Other symptoms include dysmenorrhoea, deep dyspareunia, and infertility, all of which can have an impact on the physical, mental, and social wellbeing of these women.

How common is it?

Endometriosis is estimated to affect 5-10% of women in the reproductive age group.[1] Prevalence is difficult to determine due to difficulties in diagnosis caused by the diversity of symptoms and their severity and because endometriosis may be asymptomatic.

Why is it missed?

Endometriosis is often labelled "the missed disease"[2]; in the United Kingdom the average time between onset of symptoms and a definitive diagnosis is 7-8 years.[3] This delay is usually due to failure to recognise the nature of the symptoms of endometriosis. Diagnosing the condition on the basis of symptoms alone can be difficult as they are so variable (table) [4 5 6 7] and overlap considerably with those of other conditions, such as irritable bowel syndrome and pelvic inflammatory disease, even though it is rare to isolate a microbe causing pelvic inflammatory disease from the genital tracts of women undergoing investigation of symptoms.

Diagnosis is problematic in primary care for several reasons. Patients initially present to the general practitioner not with endometriosis but with symptoms that are difficult to differentiate from other conditions. Often, women (not uncommonly soon after menarche) who present with symptoms associated with menstruation, however severe, are told that it is part of being a woman or it is just painful periods, and that they will have to bear it.[8] Many women with endometriosis are therefore mislabelled as having idiopathic dysmenorrhoea or as having pelvic inflammatory disease even when there may be no preceding episode of acute pelvic inflammatory disease. Thus the non-specific nature of symptoms may make diagnosis problematic in primary care.

KEY POINTS

- Consider a diagnosis of endometriosis in every woman of reproductive age presenting with menstrual or chronic pelvic pain, especially pain associated with dyspareunia
- All adolescents with chronic pelvic pain (especially cyclical pain) that is unresponsive to conventional treatment should be investigated for endometriosis
- The combination of pelvic tenderness, retroversion of the uterus, and induration in the posterior fornix indicates a high likelihood of endometriosis
- Where there is a strong clinical suspicion of the diagnosis in primary care, a three month trial of gonadotrophin releasing hormone agonist or the combined pill may be used to help diagnosis

Symptoms of endometriosis

Symptom	% of women with endometriosis presenting with symptom*
Dysmenorrhoea[4 5]	40-87
Bloating[4]	42
Lethargy[4]	40
Chronic pelvic pain[4 6]	20-80
Constipation[4]	29
Low back pain[4 5]	29
Deep dyspareunia[4 5]	19-42
Dyschezia[4-6]	13-30
Infertility[5]	9
Cyclical rectal bleeding[5]	9
Menorrhagia[4]	7
Diarrhoea[4]	8
Haematuria[5]	3

**Studies comprised 50 participants,[4] 101 participants,[5] and 141 participants[6]; see also the epidemiological review.[7]*

Why does this matter?

Endometriosis causes chronic pelvic pain, menstrual disorders, and infertility. A survey in 2005 showed that in the European Union, endometriosis cost member states more than €30bn a year in lost working days, and of the 7025 women with endometriosis who completed the survey, 82% reported that the condition had caused them to take time off work in the past five years.[9] About 30-40% of women with infertility have endometriosis. It is a major contributor to depression from chronic pelvic pain syndrome and to sexual dysfunction and its consequences, including relationship disharmony, bowel and bladder symptoms, and depression (from chronic pelvic pain).[10] Consequently it is not unusual for women with these symptoms to be passed from one specialist to another.

How is it diagnosed?

Clinical features

The clinical presentation of women with endometriosis varies considerably, with a significant proportion of those with the condition being asymptomatic and diagnosed incidentally at laparoscopy. Symptoms typically develop as early as adolescence and persist after menopause in some women.[11 12] Endometriosis should be considered in adolescents with chronic pelvic pain that is not responding to conventional treatment; up to 69% have endometriosis at laparosocopy.[11]

The clinical manifestation of endometriosis is diverse.[13] Case series and cohort studies show that some symptoms are more commonly reported than others (see table).[4 5 6 7] Bowel or bladder symptoms in some patients make the diagnosis difficult to distinguish from irritable bowel syndrome or interstitial cystitis.[14]

A pelvic examination may be entirely normal but classic findings include uterine and adnexal tenderness, a fixed retroverted uterus, nodularity of the uterosacral ligaments, and adnexal masses. The tenderness often makes eliciting the other classic features difficult. There is, however, evidence that performing the examination during menstruation helps to make the diagnosis, but many women will be reluctant to be examined at this time.[14]

Investigations

The indicative diagnostic test is visualisation of the pelvis at laparoscopy by an experienced gynaecologist.[3] A positive result increases the likelihood of detecting the disease histologically to 31% (95% CI 21% to 46%) and a negative result decreases the likelihood of detecting endometriosis to 0.7% (0.1% to 5.0%).[15] However, attempts should be made to reach a diagnosis on the basis of history and a detailed clinical examination rather than delaying this until a laparoscopy is performed. A therapeutic trial with gonadotrophin releasing

CASE SCENARIO

A 26 year old presents with several years of severe dysmenorrhoea (with little relief from non-steroidal anti-inflammatory drugs) and dyspareunia which is increasingly affecting her relationship with her partner. Her general practitioner suspects endometriosis, as endocervical swabs show no evidence of infection and her symptoms improve slightly after he advises her to take the pill continuously. He refers her to a gynaecologist with interest in endometriosis for more definitive management of her symptoms. Laparoscopy confirms the diagnosis and she is successfully managed with a gonadotrophin releasing hormone agonist pill for six months.

hormone agonist or the combined oral contraceptive pill (without the pill-free interval) for three months in suspected cases may also be used to help diagnosis. Ultrasound has been shown in a systematic review to be useful in diagnosing endometriomas and deep infiltrating rectovaginal disease, with a positive likelihood ratio of 7.6-29.8 and a negative likelihood ratio of 0.12-0.4.[16] Magnetic resonance imaging is of limited value in diagnosing any peritoneal disease.

How is it treated?

Although there has been much clinical research on the nature of endometriosis and on treatment alternatives, the treatment options (medical or surgical) depend on the informed choice of the woman as well as her age, fertility plans, previous treatment, the nature and severity of symptoms, and the location and severity of disease.

Medical treatment may reduce symptoms in 80-90% of patients, but none of the options has been shown to reduce recurrence of symptoms once treatment has stopped. Suppression of ovarian function for at least six months is the basis for most medical treatment, and the options include the combined oral contraceptive pill, medroxyporogesterone acetate, and gonadotrophin releasing hormone agonist.[13] More recently, the levonorgestrel intrauterine system (Mirena) has been shown to be effective even after three years of use.[17] In a small uncontrolled trial, the levonorgestrel intrauterine system (Mirena) seemed to control symptoms effectively in mild to moderate disease even after three years of use, although discontinuation rates were high.[17] Recurrence (from soon to up to three years after stopping treatment) of symptoms varies from an estimated 37% for mild disease to 74% in severe disease.[1]

The success and the advisability of surgery depends on the severity of the disease, its location, and the extent of the symptoms. Surgical options include removing entire lesions that are severe and deeply infiltrating (which may reduce pain related to endometriosis); ovarian cystectomy in the case of endometriomas; adhesiolysis; and bilateral oophorectomy, often with a hysterectomy. Patients undergoing radical surgery should be counselled about the possibility of symptoms persisting after bilateral oophorectomy.[2]

Multidisciplinary treatment should include pain management services, clinical psychologists, gynaecologists in secondary care, and general practitioners in primary care. Although centres of excellence are being advocated, these should ideally be managing advanced disease.

Contributors: SE and JCK researched and wrote the draft paper; CG contributed to the writing. JCK wrote the final version and is guarantor.

Funding: No external funding.

Competing interests: JCK has an ongoing research programme funded by Bayer on the use Mirena and decapeptyl in the management of symptoms of endometriosis.

Provenance and peer review: Commissioned; externally peer reviewed.

Patient consent not required (patient anonymised, dead, or hypothetical).

1 Winkel CA. Evaluation and management of women with endometriosis. *Obstet Gynaecol* 2003;102:397-408.
2 Royal College of Obstetricians and Gynaecologists. The investigation and management of endometriosis. 2007. www.rcog.org.uk/womens-health/clinical-guidance/investigation-and-management-endometriosis-green-top-24
3 Endometriosis.org. Endometriosis still takes 8 years to diagnose – and treatment options remain largely ineffective [press release]. 15 September 2005. www.endometriosis.org/press15september05.html
4 Louden SF, Wingfield M, Read PA, Louden KA. The incidence of atypical symptoms in patients with endometriosis. *J Obstet Gynaecol* 1995;15:307-10.
5 Meurs-Szojda MM, Mijatovic V, Felt-Bersma RJF, Hompes PGA. Irritable bowel syndrome and chronic constipation in patients with endometriosis. *Colorectal Dis* 2009 Oct 13.
6 Carter JE. Combined hysteroscopic and laparoscopic findings in patients with chronic pelvic pain. *J Am Assoc Gynecol Laparosc* 1994;2:43-7.
7 Cramer DW, Missmer SA. The epidemiology of endometriosis. *Ann N Y Acad Sci* 2002;955:11-22.
8 Barnard A. Endometriosis and pain. In: McClean AB, Stones RW, Thornton S, eds. *Pain in obstetrics and gynaecology* . London: RCOG Press, 2001:145-51.
9 European Network on Endometriosis. Introduction. www.endonetwork.eu
10 Ballard KD, Seaman HE, de Vries CS, Wright JT. Can symptomatology help in the diagnosis of endometriosis? Findings from a national case control study—part 1. *BJOG* 2008;115:1382-91.
11 Laufer MR, Goiten L, Bush M, Cramer DW, Emans SJ. Prevalence of endometriosis in adolescent girls with chronic pelvic pain not responding to conventional therapy. *J Pediatr Adolesc Gynecol* 1997;10:199-202.
12 Rosa-e-Silva JC, Carvalho BR, Barbosa Hde F, Poli-Neto OB, Rosa-e-Silva AC, Candido-dos-Reis FJ, et al. Endometriosis in postmenopausal women without previous hormonal therapy: report of three cases. *Climacteric* 2008;11:525-8.
13 Kennedy S, Bergqvist A, Chapron C, D'Hooghe T, Dunselman G, Greb R, et al. ESHRE guidelines for the diagnosis and treatment of endometriosis. *Hum Rep* 2005;20:2698-704.
14 NHS Evidence – women's health: Annual Evidence Update on Endometriosis – Clinical features and diagnosis. http://www.library.nhs.uk//womenshealth/ViewResource.aspx?resID=307263
15 Wykes CB, Clark TJ, Khan KS. Accuracy of laparoscopy in the diagnosis of endometriosis: a systematic quantitative review. *BJOG* 2004;111:1204-12.
16 Moore J, Copley S, Morris J, Lindsell D, Golding S, Kennedy S. A systematic review of the accuracy of ultrasound in the diagnosis of endometriosis. *Ultrasound Obstet Gynaecol* 2002;20:630-4.
17 Lockhat FB, Emembolu JO, Konje JC. The efficacy, side-effects and continuation rates in women with symptomatic endometriosis undergoing treatment with an intra-uterine administered progestogen (levonorgestrel): a 3 year follow-up. *Hum Reprod* 2005;20:789-93.

Lichen sclerosus

Kate Dalziel, honorary consultant dermatologist[1],
Sarah Shaw, general practitioner[2]

[1]Royal Cornwall Hospital, Truro TR1 3LJ

[2]Stennack Surgery, St Ives

Correspondence to: K Dalziel kate.dalziel@rcht.cornwall.nhs.uk

Cite this as: BMJ 2010;340:c731

DOI: 10.1136/bmj.c731

www.bmj.com/content/340/bmj.c731

Lichen sclerosus is a chronic inflammatory skin disease usually involving the anogenital skin. It is most common in postmenopausal women but occurs in both sexes at all ages.[1] The cause is unknown, but lichen sclerosus is strongly associated with autoimmune disorders, particularly thyroid disease, in almost 30% of patients.[2]

Why is it missed?

Lack of familiarity with the condition and failure to examine the genital skin properly can lead to long delays in diagnosis. Reticence and embarrassment on the part of patient and doctor may hinder the taking of a full history and examination. Common mistaken diagnoses in women are candida infection and postmenopausal vulval atrophy. Candida vulvovaginitis is usually confined to women of childbearing years[5] and is unusual in older women unless there are additional risk factors such as diabetes. The delay to diagnosis in one case series of 327 female patients was 2.2 years in children and 5.3 years in adults.[6]

Lack of familiarity with the condition probably explains why lichen sclerosus is rarely diagnosed as a cause of severe constipation in girls.[7] Terminology has been confusing in the past, when terms such as vulval dystrophy and balanitis xerotica obliterans have been used instead of lichen sclerosus. The introduction of internationally agreed terminology[8] and the advent of multidisciplinary vulval clinics have improved the recognition of lichen sclerosus and the use of correct nomenclature.

Why does this matter?

Lichen sclerosus is highly symptomatic. Vulval, penile, and perianal disease can cause severe intractable itching and soreness. Scarring may follow, leading to loss of vulval anatomy (fig 1), clitoral phimosis, and vulval stenosis in women.[1] Sexual function may be severely impaired.[9] Phimosis and anterior urethral obstruction can occur in men and boys. The development of squamous cell carcinoma on genital lichen sclerosus is a well recognised complication in both sexes and is estimated to occur in about 5% of women. Sexual abuse is sometimes suspected in children with lichen sclerosus and, although the condition does not exclude abuse, which must always be considered, this has led to mistaken diagnosis.[10]

KEY POINTS

- Always examine postmenopausal women with vulval itching for lichen sclerosus and other itchy skin disorders
- Consider lichen sclerosus in girls with severe constipation and in boys with phimosis
- Lichen sclerosus is often diagnosed by the clinical appearance, but if uncertainty exists then it is essential that a biopsy is done before very potent topical steroids are used
- Check thyroid function, and remember that a patient with lichen sclerosus is also more likely to have other autoimmune disorders
- Consider using topical steroids to treat phimosis caused by lichen sclerosus as this may avoid the need for circumcision
- Advise patients about the small (5%) risk of malignant change and to report immediately any change, such as an ulcer or lump

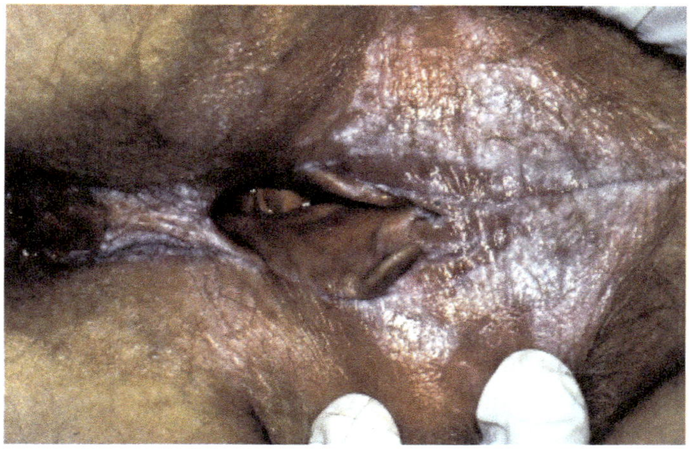

Fig 1 Vulval lichen sclerosus showing white plaques and scarring with loss of the labia minora

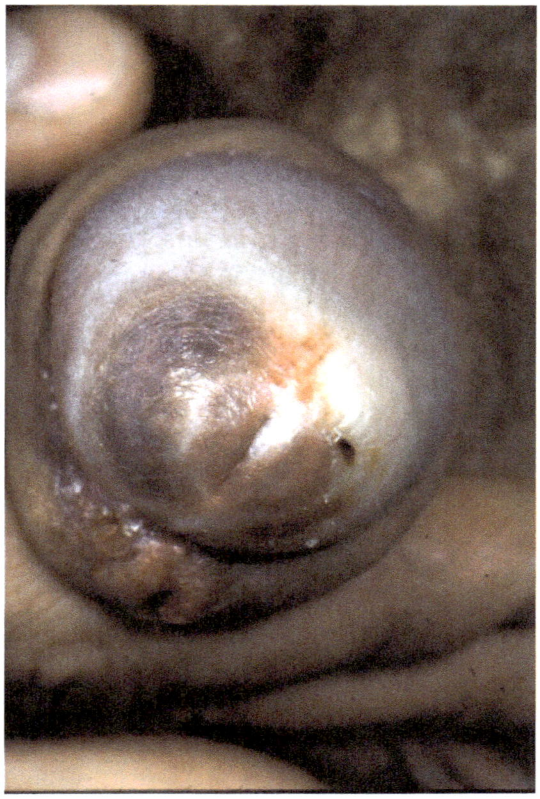

Fig 2 Lichen sclerosus of glans penis in adult showing whiteness and purpura

How is it diagnosed?

Clinical features

Adult women

The commonest presenting symptom of lichen sclerosus is severe vulval itching, and many patients will already have self medicated with over the counter anticandidal or anti-itch creams. Typical changes of lichen sclerosus include areas of white skin that may be small and numerous or confluent over larger areas affecting the labia minora, labia majora, and adjacent skin of the perineum and groin creases. Perianal disease is common, giving a "figure of eight" pattern of affected skin around the vulva and perianal region. The white skin often looks thin, wrinkled and fragile, with red or purple areas of bleeding into the skin. Excoriations are common. Sometimes there are thickened plaques or even warty areas. In a series of 253 women with lichen sclerosus, 177 had atrophic change and 94 had hyperkeratotic (warty) areas.[6]

In the patients with scarring (about 70% of women)[6] symptoms can include difficulty in passing urine, especially in men, and in women, dyspareunia, apareunia and splitting of the skin on attempted intercourse. Women may notice the change in their vulva with loss of the labia minora (fig 1) and fusion of the labia over the clitoris. Occasionally the first presentation of lichen sclerosus will be when squamous carcinoma develops: a plaque, ulcer or nodule can arise and enlarge very quickly, sometimes in a matter of weeks.

Adult men
Itching and soreness of the glans and prepuce are common. White areas and purpura can be seen on the glans and foreskin but may be hidden by a tight phimosis (fig 2). Squamous cell carcinoma can arise in the affected area, with features similar to those described above for women.

Children
Prepubertal girls with lichen sclerosus often present with vulval and perianal itching and show the typical skin changes as described for adult women, but they may also present with intractable constipation, soiling, anal fissures, and bleeding. Boys tend to present with phimosis, and this may hide the typical skin changes.

Differential diagnosis
Other chronic itchy skin diseases need to be considered. Various types of eczema that affect the perineal and perianal areas, such as contact dermatitis and seborrhoeic eczema, are common. Another auto-immune skin condition, lichen planus, can also show a predilection for genital skin. It too may cause scarring and squamous carcinoma. Plaques of vulval intraepithelial neoplasia may be white, but the other typical features of lichen sclerosus will be absent.

Investigations
No diagnostic biochemical or immunological investigations exist, but a skin biopsy will often provide the diagnosis. The histology of lichen sclerosus is distinctive, and biopsy will help to differentiate it from other skin diseases that cause anogenital itching and scarring. However, use of a very potent topical steroid (such as clobetasol propionate) may completely correct the clinical and histological changes, so such a steroid must not be used before a definitive diagnosis is made. Accurate diagnosis is important because patients with lichen sclerosus will need follow-up and education about ongoing treatment and the risk of cancer development.

Check thyroid function in all adult patients with lichen sclerosus, given the association with autoimmune thyroid disease.

How is it managed?
Evidence based guidelines for the management of lichen sclerosus state that if clinical doubt exists then a biopsy should be performed to confirm the diagnosis.[11] The general practitioner may wish to refer the patient to a specialist with an interest in vulval disease or to an established vulval clinic (based in dermatology, genitourinary medicine, or gynaecology departments). Pending the definitive diagnosis, emollients can be used as soap substitutes and to help repair the skin barrier, and a moderate potency topical steroid such as clobetasol butyrate ointment can be used sparingly. After diagnosis, the accepted treatment is with the very potent topical steroid clobetasol propionate ointment.[11] No controlled trials have been published to establish the best regime, but the guidelines suggest a single application at night for four weeks followed by alternate nights for four weeks and then twice a week for four weeks. Once symptoms are well controlled, the steroid ointment is used as required. Some patients will achieve complete remission; others will require ongoing treatment. In women, surgery is reserved for correcting the effects of scarring and for removal of cancer. Surgery is not otherwise appropriate for benign disease as it is mutilating and there is rapid relapse of the lichen sclerosus.

CASE SCENARIO

An 89 year old woman presents with severe vulval itch that wakes her at night. She had previously been prescribed topical clotrimazole cream and subsequently oestrogen cream with no response.

Examination shows white plaques, areas of purpura, and excoriation of the skin around the vulva and perianal region. You suspect lichen sclerosus and refer her to the vulval clinic. You also prescribe a moderately potent topical steroid and an emollient and check her thyroid function. At the vulval clinic a diagnosis of vulval lichen sclerosus with scarring is confirmed by vulval biopsy, and very potent topical steroids are prescribed, with excellent clinical response.

HOW COMMON IS LICHEN SCLEROSUS?

- No good prevalence data exist for lichen sclerosus in either sex
- Lichen sclerosus is one of the most frequently seen conditions in vulval clinics.[1] It is the commonest underlying skin disease in elderly women presenting with squamous carcinoma of the vulva[3]
- It has been found in 60% of boys requiring circumcision for acquired phimosis[4]

In men, circumcision may sometimes be needed for phimosis. However, treatment with a very potent topical steroid may avoid the need for circumcision in both men[12] and boys.[13] In children, if the diagnosis is not certain then referral to a specialist is indicated rather than attempting a biopsy.

Useful support and advice for patients can be found on the National Lichen Sclerosus Support Group's website www.lichensclerosus.org.

Contributors: KD conceived the article and provided the background content about lichen sclerosus and its presentation and treatment. SS added the differential diagnoses as they present in general practice, the case study, and pointers to appropriate referral criteria. KD is the guarantor.

Funding: No special funding.

Competing interests: None declared.

Provenance and peer review: Not commissioned; externally peer reviewed.

Patient consent not required (patient anonymised, dead, or hypothetical).

1 Powell J, Wojnarowska F. Lichen sclerosus. *Lancet* 1999;353:1777-83.
2 Birenbaum DL, Young RC. High prevalence of thyroid disease in patients with lichen sclerosus. *J Reprod Med* 2007;52:28-30.
3 Zaki I, Dalziel KL, Solomonsz FA, Stevens A. The under-reporting of skin disease in association with squamous cell carcinoma of the vulva. *Clin Exp Dermatol* 1996;21:234-337.
4 Mattioli G, Repetto P, Carlini C, Granata C, Gambini C, Jasonni V. Lichen sclerosus et atrophicus in children with phimosis and hypospadias. *Pediatr Surg Int* 2002;18:273-5.
5 Fidel PL Jr, Cutright J, Steele C. Effects of reproductive hormones on experimental vaginal candidiasis. *Infect Immun* 2000;68:651-7.
6 Cooper SM, Gao X-H, Powell JJ, Wojnarowska F. Does treatment of vulvar lichen sclerosus influence its prognosis? *Arch Dermatol* 2004;140:702-6.
7 Maronn ML, Esterly NB. Constipation as a feature of anogenital lichen sclerosus in children. *Pediatrics* 2005;115:e230-2.
8 Lynch PJ, Moyal-Barrocco M, Bogliatto F, Micheletti L, Scurry J. 2006 ISSVD classification of vulvar dermatoses: pathologic subsets and their clinical correlates. *J Reprod Med* 2007;52:3-9.
9 Dalziel KL. Effect of lichen sclerosus on sexual function and parturition. *J Reprod Med* 1995;40:351-4.
10 Powell J, Wojnarowska F. Childhood vulvar lichen sclerosus: an increasingly common problem. *J Am Acad Dermatol* 2001;44:803-6
11 Neill SM, Tatnall FM, Cox NH. Guidelines for the management of lichen sclerosus. *Br J Dermatol* 2002;147:640-9.
12 Riddell L, Edwards A, Sherrard J. Clinical features of lichen sclerosus in men attending a department of genitourinary medicine. *Sex Transm Infect* 2000;76:311-3.
13 Jorgensen ET, Svensson A. The treatment of phimosis in boys with a potent topical steroid (clobetasol propionate 0.05%) cream. *Acta Derm Venereol* 1993;73(1):55-6.

Cholesteatoma

Mahmood F Bhutta, clinical research fellow[1], visiting scientist[2],
Ian G Williamson, clinical senior lecturer[3],
Holger H Sudhoff, professor of otolaryngology/head and neck surgery[4]

[1]Nuffield Department of Surgical Sciences (University of Oxford), John Radcliffe Hospital, Oxford OX3 9DU, UK

[2]MRC Harwell, Harwell Science and Innovation Campus, UK

[3]School of Medicine, University of Southampton, Southampton, UK

[4]Bielefeld Academic Teaching Hospital, Münster University, D-33604 Bielefeld, Germany

Correspondence to: M F Bhutta m.bhutta@doctors.org.uk

Cite this as: *BMJ* 2011;342:d1088

DOI: 10.1136/bmj.d1088

www.bmj.com/content/342/bmj.d1088

A cholesteatoma is a lesion of the ear, formed of a mass of stratified keratinising squamous epithelium (fig 1).[1] Aetiology is debated,[2] but cholesteatoma probably arises from the lateral epithelium of the tympanic membrane, and then grows as a self perpetuating mass into the middle ear. This may activate local osteoclasts,[3] possibly as a result of infection of dead epithelium at the centre of the lesion, with potentially serious consequences from local tissue destruction.

Why is cholesteatoma missed?

The onset of disease may be insidious with intermittent or mild symptoms. Typically cholesteatoma presents with intermittent unilateral otorrhoea (ear discharge) and a progressive hearing loss,[6] which may mimic and be misdiagnosed as recurrent or chronic otitis externa or otitis media. Successful negligence claims have been filed in the United Kingdom (http://boyesturnerclaims.com/case-study.html?id=85) and the United States (www.upton-hatfield.com/news/verdicts.html) for complications resulting from a missed diagnosis in primary care, although no published data are available on frequency of misdiagnosis.

Why does it matter?

A cholesteatoma is a self perpetuating mass, which if untreated, can cause extensive local tissue destruction. At presentation the ossicles are often eroded, contributing to conductive hearing loss.[7] Rarely cholesteatoma may erode into the inner ear causing sensorineural hearing loss or vertigo, or lead to facial palsy from damage to the facial nerve as it traverses the middle ear.[8] Cholesteatoma can also lead to spread of infection through the tegmen (roof) of the middle ear causing meningitis or intracranial abscess (fig 2), a risk estimated to be 1 in 10 000 a year of untreated disease.[9]

How is cholesteatoma diagnosed?

Clinical features

Symptoms of cholesteatoma—such as persistent hearing loss (present in 83% of 23 ears in a case series), otorrhoea (56%), otalgia (39%), vertigo, or tinnitus—are non-specific,[6] and so the diagnosis rests on the appearance on otoscopic examination. Cholesteatoma is classically described as "wax in the attic": a yellow or white crust visible in the upper part (pars flaccida or "attic") of the tympanic membrane, often surrounded by pus and with a perforation of the adjacent tympanic membrane and erosion of the surrounding bone (fig 1). In advanced cases, bony erosion may be severe and normal anatomy difficult to recognise. Whereas most cholesteatomas arise in the attic, they can also arise in the lower part (pars tensa) of the tympanic membrane.[7]

KEY POINTS

- Cholesteatoma is a locally destructive lesion of the middle ear, in the form of a cyst of keratinous epithelium
- Cholesteatoma can occasionally lead to serious consequences, including facial palsy, meningitis, or brain abscess
- It should be suspected in any case of persistent or recurrent ear discharge
- The key to diagnosis is a characteristic appearance on otoscopy

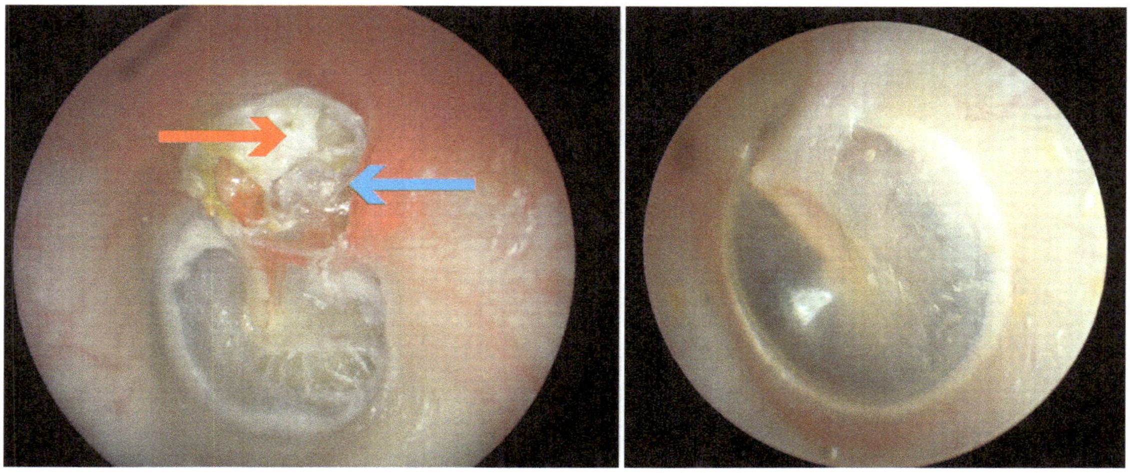

Fig 1 Left: Cholesteatoma (red arrow) arising in the upper part (pars flaccida or "attic") of left tympanic membrane. Note erosion of surrounding bone (blue arrow). Right: Normal tympanic membrane (left ear) for comparison

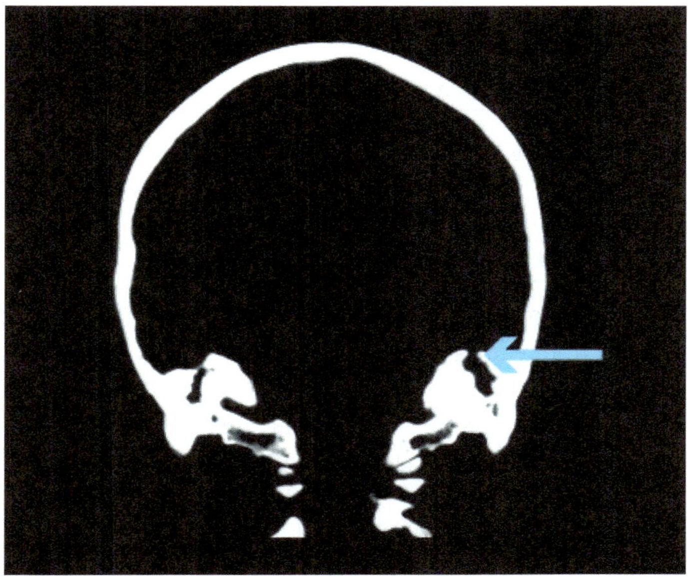

Fig 2 Sagittal computed tomogram through the temporal bones of a patient with longstanding left cholesteatoma. The bony tegmen (roof) of the left middle ear has eroded (arrow), leading to an abscess in the temporal lobe

In primary care, cholesteatoma should be suspected in an ear with recurrent or persistent otorrhoea that fails to settle fully with treatment. In general practice such symptoms are more often the result of recurrent otitis externa or recurrent otitis media,[10] but only a full visualisation of the tympanic membrane allows cholesteatoma to be excluded. In all new cases of facial palsy otoscopy should be used to exclude cholesteatoma as a cause.[11]

Visualisation, however, may be difficult. When a cholesteatoma is temporarily or permanently active, the external auditory canal may become filled with purulent discharge and be oedematous, and if facilities are not available for aural toilet, obtaining an adequate view of the tympanic membrane may be impossible. Chronic inflammation may also cause the formation of a macroscopic polyp of granulation tissue,[12] which again can obstruct the view. In paediatric cases the child may not permit examination. In difficult cases it is worth treating the ear for a presumed infection and bringing the patient back for re-examination of the ear once infection has settled. When visualisation is still difficult and symptoms continue, refer the patient to an otolaryngologist for aural toilet or application of topical steroid creams to granulation tissue (possibly under general anaesthesia for a child); this

CASE SCENARIO

A 24 year old man presented to his general practitioner several times over a year with an intermittently discharging left ear and associated hearing loss. Visualisation of the tympanic membrane was not possible owing to otorrhoea and oedema in the external auditory canal. He was treated for presumed otitis externa with repeated courses of topical antibiotic drops, but as improvement was only temporary he was referred to a specialist. An otolaryngologist cleared the external auditory canal of debris ("aural toilet") and discovered a cholesteatoma arising from the left tympanic membrane; this was successfully treated by surgical excision.

HOW COMMON IS CHOLESTEATOMA?

- The estimated incidence of cholesteatoma in northern Europe is 9.2 per 100000 population a year[4]
- Therefore a general practitioner with a practice size of 2500 patients would be expected to see on average one new case every four to five years
- The peak incidence is in the age range 5-15 years,[5] but cholesteatoma can arise in any age group
- Seven per cent of people diagnosed will subsequently develop cholesteatoma in the contralateral ear[5]
- The incidence is reportedly higher in white than non-white populations

will allow the tympanic membrane to be seen and the presence or absence of cholesteatoma verified.

Investigations

High resolution computed tomography can help to define the likely extent of a cholesteatoma, and it may show bony erosion, which makes the diagnosis more likely.[13] It may also show complications from more advanced disease. Diffusion weighted magnetic resonance imaging has also been used to show cholesteatoma.[14] However, no imaging is sufficiently sensitive or specific for cholesteatoma,[15] and the cornerstone of diagnosis remains clinical, based on the appearance on otoscopy.

An audiogram is needed to define the degree and type of hearing loss. Typically a conductive hearing loss is found, as a result of the cholesteatoma mass itself or erosion of ossicles, but an additional sensorineural hearing loss may be present if the cochlea has also sustained damage.

How is it managed?

When cholesteatoma is diagnosed or suspected, "semi-urgent" referral (for the patient to be seen by a specialist within a few weeks) is appropriate. However, if facial palsy is also present, refer immediately, because if the palsy is caused by the cholesteatoma, delayed treatment is associated with a worse prognosis.[16 17 18] The presence of pain or other neurological symptoms or signs should also prompt urgent referral as these may portend intracranial complications.

Surgical excision is the only known cure for cholesteatoma, and the choice of operation depends on the extent of the lesion. Local excision may be sufficient for early cholesteatoma, but more extensive disease requires exploration of the mastoid air cells with a mastoidectomy. This sometimes means that the mastoid air cells are "externalised" by surgical excision of the posterior external auditory canal, to form a mastoid cavity. The risk of residual disease after surgery varies (5% to 30%) with the procedure and extent of the disease, and patients require follow-up and sometimes repeat exploratory surgery.

In some older patients and in patients with concurrent morbidity, conservative management of cholesteatoma may be an option, but as highlighted above, this carries a small but continuing risk of serious complications from this disease.

Thanks to David Pothier for providing the images in figure 1.

Contributors: MFB conceptualised the article and researched and wrote the first draft. IGW and HHS made important revisions.

Funding: No additional funding.

Competing interests: All authors have completed the Unified Competing Interest form at www.icmje.org/coi_disclosure.pdf (available on request from the corresponding author) and declare: no support from any company for the submitted work; IGW has previously received an honorarium from GlaxoSmithKline for a symposium on prescribing in otitis media; and no non-financial interests that may be relevant to the submitted work.

Provenance and peer review: Not commissioned; externally peer reviewed.

Patient consent not required (patient anonymised, dead, or hypothetical).

1 Browning GG, Merchant SM, Kelly G, Swan IRC, Canter R, McKerrow WS. Chronic otitis media. In: Gleeson MJ, ed. *Scott-Brown's otorhinolaryngology, head and neck surgery* . 7th ed. Hodder Arnold, 2008:3395-445.

2 Olszewska E, Wagner M, Bernal-Sprekelsen M, Ebmeyer J, Dazert S, Hildmann H, et al. Etiopathogenesis of cholesteatoma. *Eur Arch Otorhinolaryngol* 2004;261(1):6-24.

3 Jung JY, Chole RA. Bone resorption in chronic otitis media: the role of the osteoclast. *ORL J Otorhinolaryngol Relat Spec* 2002;64:95-107.

4 Kemppainen HO, Puhakka HJ, Laippala PJ, Sipila MM, Manninen MP, Karma PH. Epidemiology and aetiology of middle ear cholesteatoma. *Acta Otolaryngol* 1999;119:568-72.

5 Rosenfeld RM, Moura RL, Bluestone CD. Predictors of residual-recurrent cholesteatoma in children. *Arch Otolaryngol Head Neck Surg* 1992;118:384-91.

6 Sheahan P, Donnelly M, Kane R. Clinical features of newly presenting cases of chronic otitis media. *J Laryngol Otol* 2001;115:962-6.

7 Wetmore RF, Konkle DF, Potsic WP, Handler SD. Cholesteatoma in the pediatric patient. *Int J Pediatr Otorhinolaryngol* 1987;14:101-12.

8 Smith JA, Danner CJ. Complications of chronic otitis media and cholesteatoma. *Otolaryngol Clin North Am* 2006;39:1237-55.

9 Nunez DA, Browning GG. Risks of developing an otogenic intracranial abscess. *J Laryngol Otol* 1990;104:468-72.

10 Bain J, Williamson I. Treating the discharging ear in general practice. *BMJ* 1988;296:1617.

11 Syed I, Bhutta M. Facial nerve palsy: assessment and management. *Br J Hosp Med (Lond)* 2008;69(3):M34-7.

12 Milroy CM, Slack RW, Maw AR, Bradfield JW. Aural polyps as predictors of underlying cholesteatoma. *J Clin Pathol* 1989;42:460-5.

13 Lemmerling MM, de Foer B, VandeVyver V, Vercruysse JP, Verstraete KL. Imaging of the opacified middle ear. *Eur J Radiol* 2008;66:363-71.

14 Vercruysse JP, de Foer B, Somers T, Casselman J, Offeciers E. Magnetic resonance imaging of cholesteatoma: an update. *B-ENT* 2009;5:233-40.

15 O'Reilly BJ, Chevretton EB, Wylie I, Thakkar C, Butler P, Sathanathan N, et al. The value of CT scanning in chronic suppurative otitis media. *J Laryngol Otol* 1991;105:990-4.

16 Omran A, De Denato G, Piccirillo E, Leone O, Sanna M. Petrous bone cholesteatoma: management and outcomes. *Laryngoscope* 2006;116:619-26.

17 Ikeda M, Nakazato H, Onoda K, Hirai R, Kida A. Facial nerve paralysis caused by middle ear cholesteatoma and effects of surgical intervention. *Acta Otolaryngol* 2006;126:95-100.

18 Siddiq MA, Hanu-Cernat LM, Irving RM. Facial palsy secondary to cholesteatoma: analysis of outcome following surgery. *J Laryngol Otol* 2007;121:114-7.

BPP UNIVERSITY SCHOOL OF HEALTH BMJ

Giant cell arteritis

Nada Hassan, specialist registrar[1],
Bhaskar Dasgupta, consultant rheumatologist[1],
Kevin Barraclough, general practitioner[2]

[1]Rheumatology, Southend University Hospital, Westcliff-on-Sea SSo oRY, UK

[2]Greenbank, Painswick GL6 6TY, UK

Correspondence to: K Barraclough k.barraclough@btinternet.com

Cite this as: *BMJ* 2011;342:d3019

DOI: 10.1136/bmj.d3019

www.bmj.com/content/342/bmj.d3019

Giant cell arteritis affects large and medium sized arteries, often branches of the external carotid artery but also the ciliary and retinal arteries. The symptoms are caused by local ischaemia due to endovascular damahge and cytokine mediated systemic illness. There is considerable overlap with polymyalgia rheumatica: 16-21% of patients with polymyalgia rheumatica have giant cell arteritis on temporal artery biopsy, and symptoms of polymyalgia rheumatica are present in 40-60% of patients with giant cell arteritis.[1]

Why is giant cell arteritis missed?

A systematic review analysed the presenting clinical features in a mixture of studies with a total of 1435 cases of giant cell arteritis.[3] The sensitivity of individual clinical features was relatively low (table), reflecting the diverse presentation of this condition: 24% of cases had no headache at all, and only 52% had a temporal headache. Giant cell arteritis can be easily missed when systemic symptoms (such as low grade fever or weight loss), ischaemic symptoms (jaw claudication or transient visual symptoms), or polymyalgic symptoms (proximal myalgia or morning stiffness) predominate over the well known hallmark of temporal headache. The mean duration of symptoms in the 1435 patients at diagnosis was 3.5 months. A 1971 Swedish study examined 1097 consecutive autopsies with temporal artery examination carried out in each of them. Sixteen cases of undiagnosed giant cell arteritis were identified. Retrospective analysis of the case notes documented typical features of undiagnosed giant cell arteritis in 9.[4] A recent audit of 65 patients with giant cell arteritis showed that 44 had had unrecognised visual disturbance, visual loss or stroke in the mean of 35 days between onset of symptoms and diagnosis (range of 2 to 336 days).[5] Eleven of these patients presented without headache or scalp tenderness and 10 of these had visual loss.

Why does this matter?

Acute blindness occurs in up to 20% of patients with giant cell arteritis.[4] Delay in recognition may explain the high incidence of irreversible loss of vision, which is preventable with early diagnosis and treatment.[4] Jaw or tongue claudication occurs in a minority of cases but heralds a high rsik of impending ischaemic complications.[6]

LEARNING POINTS

- Giant cell arteritis is a medical emergency, as irreversible loss of vision can occur in 20% of cases without prompt treatment with steroids
- "Typical" features such as headache and scalp tenderness may be absent, and this subgroup has a high risk of visual loss
- Jaw or tongue claudication occurs in a minority of cases and heralds impending ischaemic complications
- Erythrocyte sedimentation rate and C-reactive protein are normal in only 4% of cases but may be just mildly raised in a fifth of cases
- If giant cell arteritis is suspected, immediate treatment with high dose corticosteroids is indicated, and temporal biopsy should be arranged within two weeks of starting treatment

Sensitivity of clinical features in predicting giant cell arteritis[3]

Clinical feature	% of biopsy proven cases (sensitivity)
Headache:	
Any headache	76
Temporal headache	52
Scalp tenderness	31
Jaw claudication	34
Visual symptoms:	
Any visual symptom	37
Unilateral visual loss	24
Diplopia	9
Myalgia	39
Previous diagnosis of polymyalgia rheumatica	34
Weight loss	43
Fever	42
Temporal artery:	
Pulse absent	45
Any abnormality on palpation of temporal artery (absent, prominent, beaded)	65
Erythrocyte sedimentation rate:	
"Normal"	4
>50 mm/h	83

How is giant cell arteritis diagnosed?

The typical presentation of giant cell arteritis is with temporal headache of recent onset, myalgia, or systemic malaise or fever, and the mean age of onset is 70. Erythrocyte sedimentation rate or C reactive protein is typically raised.[2] The case presented illustrates that "typical" features may be absent or subtle.

A meta-analysis looked at studies examining the value of individual clinical features in predicting positive results of temporal artery biopsy in patients with suspected giant cell arteritis.[3] No clinical features had a high negative likelihood ratio, because no clinical feature (even headache) was reliably present in all cases. Several symptoms were moderately predictive of a positive biopsy result (likelihood ratio >2):

- Jaw claudication (present in 34% of cases); claudicant pain comes on gradually during chewing, whereas temperomandibular pain or dental pain is immediate
- Diplopia (present 8% of cases)
- Any abnormality on palpation of the temporal artery—absent, beaded, tender, or enlarged (present in 65% of cases).

Other useful predictive features (likelihood ratio >1.5) were

- Temporal headache
- Scalp tenderness
- Erythrocyte sedimentation rate >100 mm/h
- Anaemia.

The limitation of these studies is that giant cell arteritis was already highly likely, as all patients in the studied population had biopsies. In practice, the condition should be suspected in anyone over the age of 50 with headache, scalp tenderness, transient visual symptoms, or unexplained facial pain. Examination may show no abnormalities, but palpation of the temporal artery is often abnormal. Only 4% of patients have a completely "normal" erythrocyte sedimentation rate (half the age of the patient, plus 5 for women[7]); 83% have a rate above 50 mm/h.Once giant cell arteritis is suspected, refer patients urgently for temporal artery biopsy, which needs to be done within two weeks of starting steroids.

CASE SCENARIO

A previously fit and well 72 year old man presented to his general practitioner after several months of malaise and weight loss. When asked about any pain, he pointed to his left scalp as being painful. Examination was normal except that his left temporal artery was not palpable. Suspecting giant cell arteritis, the GP started 40 mg prednisolone and requested an erythrocyte sedimentation rate, which was 86 mm/h. The symptoms largely disappeared in 48 hours. She also referred the patient for a temporal artery biopsy, which showed giant cell arteritis.

HOW COMMON IS IT?

- Giant cell arteritis occurs in 2.2 per 10000 patient years in the United Kingdom[2]
- A full time general practitioner may expect to see one new case every 1-2 years
- It is virtually unknown in people aged under 50

The true sensitivity of temporal biopsy is not known, but one model estimates a sensitivity of 87%.[8]

How is giant cell arteritis managed?

Most treatment recommendations are based on experts' opinion, as randomised trials would be unethical.[7] Once the diagnosis is suspected, treat with high dose corticosteroid immediately. Give 40 mg prednisolone daily unless the patient has ischaemic symptoms (jaw or tongue claudication, or visual symptoms). With claudication symptoms, give 60 mg prednisolone daily; if the patient has visual symptoms, admit for treatment with intravenous methylprednisolone.Once symptoms and abnormal test results resolve, the dose can be reduced in 10 mg steps each two weeks to 20 mg, then in 2.5 mg steps. Most patients have stopped taking steroids by two years.[9]

Contributors: KB conceived the idea. NH and BD wrote the first draft; KB revised it. All authors approved the article before publication. KB is guarantor.

Funding: No additional funding.

Competing interests: All authors have completed the Unified Competing Interest form at www.icmje.org/coi_disclosure.pdf and declare: no support from any organisation for the submitted work; no financial relationships with any organisations that might have an interest in the submitted work in the previous three years. KB and BD were authors of the 2010 British Society of Rheumatologists guidelines on the management of giant cell arteritis.

Provenance and peer review: Not commissioned; externally peer reviewed.

Patient consent not required (patient anonymised, dead, or hypothetical).

1 Salvarani C, Cantini F, Hunder GG. Polymyalgia rheumatica and giant-cell arteritis. *Lancet* 2008;372:234-45.
2 Smeeth L, Cook C, Hall AJ. Incidence of diagnosed polymyalgia rheumatica and temporal arteritis in the United Kingdom, 1990 to 2001. *Ann Rheum Dis* 2006;65:1093-8.
3 Smetana GW, Shmerling RH. Does this patient have temporal arteritis? *JAMA* 2002;287:92-101.
4 Ostberg G. Temporal arteritis in a large necropsy series. *Ann Rheum Dis* 1971;30:224-35.
5 Ezeonyeji AN, Borg FA, Dasgupta B. Delays in recognition and management of giant cell arteritis: results from a retrospective audit. *Clin Rheumatol* 2011;30:259-62.
6 Salvarni C, Cimino L, Macchioni P, Consonni D, Cantinni F, Bajocchi G, et al. Risk factors for visual loss in an Italian population-based cohort of patients with giant cell arteritis. *Arthritis Rheum* 2005;53:293-7.
7 Miller A, Green M, Robinson D. Simple rule for calculating normal erythrocyte sedimentation rate. *BMJ* 1983;286:266.
8 Niederkohr RD, Levin LA. A Bayesian analysis of the true sensitivity of a temporal artery biopsy. *Invest Opthalmol Vis Sci* 2007;48:675-80.
9 Dasgupta B, Borg FA, Hassan N, Alexander L, Barraclough K, Bourke B, et al. BSR and BHPR guidelines for the management of giant cell arteritis. *Rheumatology* 2010;keq039a.

Kawasaki disease

Anthony Harnden, professor of primary care[1],
Robert Tulloh, professor of congenital cardiology[2],
David Burgner, professor[3]

[1]Department of Primary Care Health Sciences, University of Oxford, Oxford, UK

[2]University Hospitals Bristol NHS Foundation Trust, University of Bristol, Bristol, UK

[3]Murdoch Childrens Research Institute and Department of Paediatrics, University of Melbourne, Parkville, VIC, Australia

Correspondence to: anthony.harnden@phc.ox.ac.uk

Cite this as: *BMJ* 2014;349:g5336

DOI: 10.1136/bmj.g5336

http://www.bmj.com/content/349/bmj.g5336

Case scenario

A 2 year old boy was brought to see the general practitioner by his parents because of a four day history of fever. His parents noticed a rash and slightly "bloodshot" eyes the day before. The GP diagnosed a viral illness, offered reassurance, but gave good safety netting advice. The boy re-presented to his GP three days later, still intermittently febrile, irritable, and with an angry looking widespread morbilliform rash and a sore mouth. Kawasaki disease was suspected, and he was admitted to hospital where he received prompt treatment with intravenous immunoglobulin and high dose aspirin. An echocardiogram, performed during admission was normal, as were those during follow-up.

What is Kawasaki disease?

Kawasaki disease is an acute inflammatory vasculitis of medium size arteries that occurs mainly in children aged 6 months to 5 years but can occur at any age, including younger infants, and even occasionally in adults.[1 2 3] Although one or multiple infectious triggers are most likely, the precise cause is unclear. Kawasaki disease is the commonest cause of acquired heart disease in children in industrialised countries because the coronary arteries are affected in about a quarter of untreated cases. The incidence of acquired heart disease in children is rising.[4]

Why is Kawasaki disease missed?

A recent observational study of Kawasaki disease set in primary care reported a delay of more than 10 days (range of the time for the total sample between GP presentation and admission was 0-86 days) between first presentation and hospital admission for 7% of children.[11] In the initial stages the fever and rash of Kawasaki disease can mimic viral exanthemata, such as parvovirus, adenovirus, and measles, as well as group A streptococcal infection. Parents might be falsely reassured that their child has a simple febrile illness and delay seeking further advice when symptoms persist or new symptoms appear. In any infant under 6 months, a prolonged fever of seven days or more, with laboratory evidence of inflammation, should be considered as Kawasaki disease and be referred for assessment and possible treatment.[12]

KEY POINTS

- Consider a diagnosis of Kawasaki disease in young children with irritability and prolonged fever (>5 days) and refer to hospital for assessment and treatment
- Incomplete Kawasaki disease—fever but fewer than four of the other diagnostic criteria (bilateral conjuntival injection, polymorphous exanthema, changes to the extremities or lips and oral cavity or both)—represents 15-20% of cases
- Treatment with intravenous immunoglobulin within five to 10 days of fever onset reduces the incidence of coronary artery lesions from 25% to ~5%
- A transthoracic echocardiogram is essential to identify coronary artery abnormalities, assess myocardial and valvular function, and exclude clinically important pericardial effusion, but a normal study does not exclude Kawasaki disease

Why does it matter?

Kawasaki disease can cause damage and dilation of the coronary arteries, including aneurysms. These may be small, but in some, there can be substantial dilation or even giant aneurysms (>8 mm internal diameter). These can thrombose acutely or can heal with stenosis, causing myocardial ischaemia many months or years later.[13] In addition, there might be acute myocarditis, leading to poor heart function, valvular regurgitation, or pericardial effusion.

It is important that Kawasaki disease is diagnosed early because treatment with intravenous immunoglobulin within five to 10 days of fever onset reduces the incidence of coronary artery lesions from 25% to ~5%.[12 13] Delays in treatment might lead to unnecessary morbidity and occasionally death. The mortality rate is about 0.2% and is most commonly secondary to thrombosis of giant aneurysms or later myocardial ischaemia and infarction.[12] Infants under 6 months, who have had fever for seven days or more, are often diagnosed late owing to incomplete features, and they might have serious, potentially life--threatening complications.[14]

How is Kawasaki disease diagnosed?

Clinical features

The diagnosis of Kawasaki disease is made on clinical grounds. Fever is universal and typically unresponsive to antipyretics and antibiotics. The diagnostic clinical criteria are individually insensitive and non-specific. Definite Kawasaki disease is characterised by prolonged fever (usually defined as .5 days) and at least four out of five key diagnostic features (box). Children with prolonged fever and suspected Kawasaki disease should be referred promptly for further assessment.

The clinical features often occur sequentially and some might have resolved by presentation, so a focused history is essential. Children who have been vaccinated with BCG might have inflammation at the vaccination site. Children with Kawasaki disease are often noticeably irritable. Incomplete Kawasaki disease (fever but less than four diagnostic criteria) is common (15-20% of all cases), so a high index of suspicion is needed for any young child or infant with prolonged fever and no clear diagnosis. Incomplete Kawasaki disease is associated with increased incidence of coronary artery abnormalities, possibly caused by delayed diagnosis.[12 14]

Investigations

No diagnostic test is available for Kawasaki disease. Laboratory features can aid the diagnosis but, as with the clinical diagnostic criteria, they lack individual specificity and sensitivity. Leucocytosis and neutrophilia are usually found. Thrombocytosis is common but occurs subacutely (week two to three), so it is not helpful diagnostically. Inflammatory markers are typically raised and mild abnormalities of liver function tests are common. White blood cells are often present in the (sterile) urine or cerebrospinal fluid, or both. A microbiologically confirmed infection is also present in a third of patients with Kawasaki disease and should not preclude the diagnosis.[15]

A transthoracic echocardiogram is essential to identify coronary artery abnormalities, assess myocardial and valvular function, and exclude a clinically important pericardial effusion. These changes might be identified at presentation in severe cases but usually develop in the subacute phase (2-3 weeks). Echocardiography is therefore not useful diagnostically, and a normal study should not influence the decision to treat Kawasaki disease. Echocardiography is performed at presentation, with follow-up echocardiograms at two weeks—if there is concern—six weeks, and often at six months. Subjective brightness of the walls of the coronary arteries, mild dilation (ectasia), or frank aneurysms might be seen.[16]

HOW COMMON IS KAWASAKI DISEASE?

- England—8.39 per 100 000 children under 5 years[5]
- Australia—9.34 per 100 000 children under 5 years[6]
- Japan—239 per 100 000 children under 5 years[7]
- Korea—134 per 100 000 children under 5 years[8]
- Taiwan—66 per 100 000 children under 5 years[9]
- Hawaii—210 per 100 000 Japanese American children under 5 years, and 13 per 100 000 white children under 5 years[10]

THE DIAGNOSTIC FEATURES OF KAWASAKI DISEASE[12]

Fever (>39°C) for at least four days and at least four of the following features, after exclusion of other similar diseases*

- Bilateral non-exudative bulbar conjunctival injection
- Polymorphous exanthema
- Changes in the extremities (acute—erythema of palms and soles, oedema of hands and feet. Subacute—periungual peeling of fingers and toes)
- Changes to lips and oral cavity (red, fissured lips, strawberry tongue, erythema of oropharyngeal mucosa, without exudates)
- Cervical lymphadenopathy (≥1.5 cm, usually unilateral, rare in infants)

How is Kawasaki disease managed?

Hospital admission is necessary. On the basis of randomised control trials, intravenous polyclonal immunoglobulin has become the established treatment, and it reduces the risk of coronary artery aneurysms from 25% to less than 5%.[12 17] Aspirin is given, although dosing regimens vary.[17 18] Additional corticosteroids have been recommended in some countries for severe and evolving cases.[17] About 15% of patients do not respond to immunoglobulin, and subsequent treatment often comprises a second infusion of immunoglobulin and intravenous methylprednisolone.[12 17 19]

Most children in industrialised countries have few long term sequelae if treated promptly and appropriately. A small proportion of children with major coronary artery damage will require ongoing specialist management. Some patients report behavioural changes and desquamation of fingers and toes with subsequent febrile illness.[20] Live vaccines (such as measles, mumps, and rubella) should be delayed for 11 months after treatment with intravenous immunoglobulin. Recurrence is rare (<1%), the risk in siblings is probably modestly increased (about 10 times the population risk in Japan).[12] Kawasaki disease is not contagious. Families of children with this disease might benefit from follow-up with a doctor familiar with the condition to allay anxiety and answer specific queries, even if there are no long term coronary artery abnormalities.

Competing interests: We have read and understood the BMJ policy on declaration of interests and declare the following interests: DB has salary and support for research into Kawasaki disease from the National Health and Medical Research Council, and Murdoch Childrens Research Institute; he also has invitations (partly reimbursed) to present Kawasaki disease-related research findings at conferences of the European Society for Paediatric Infectious Diseases, World Society for Paediatric Infectious Diseases, International Kawasaki Disease Symposia, and the World Congress of Cardiology; DB is also involved in the preparation of educational material for the Kawasaki Disease Foundation, Australia. None of these agencies or bodies had any input or influence over the manuscript at any stage. AH and RT have no interests to declare.

Provenance and peer review: not commissioned; externally peer reviewed.

Patient consent not required (patient anonymised, dead, or hypothetical).

1 Burns JC, Glodé MP. Kawasaki syndrome. *Lancet* 2004;364:533-44.
2 Harnden A, Takahashi M, Burgner D. Kawasaki disease. *BMJ* 2009;338:b1514.
3 Yim D, Curtis N, Cheung M, Burgner D. An update on Kawasaki disease II: clinical features, diagnosis, treatment and outcomes. *J Paediatr Child Health* 2013;49:614-23.
4 Yim D, Curtis N, Cheung M, Burgner D Update on Kawasaki disease: epidemiology, aetiology and pathogenesis. *J Paediatr Child Health* 2013;49:704-8.
5 Harnden A, Mayon-White R, Perera R, Yeates D, Goldacre M, Burgner D. Kawasaki disease in England: ethnicity, deprivation, and respiratory pathogens. *Pediatr Infect Dis J* 2009;28:21-4.
6 Saundankar J, Yim D, Itotoh B, Payne R, Maslin K, Jape G, et al. The epidemiology and clinical features of Kawasaki disease in Australia. *Pediatrics* 2014;133:e1009-14.
7 Nakamura Y, Yashiro M, Uehara R, Sadakane A, Tsuboi S, Aoyama, et al. Epidemiologic features of Kawasaki disease in Japan: results of the 2009-2010 nationwide survey. *J Epidemiol* 2012;22:216-21.
8 Kim GB, Han JW, Park YW, Song MS, Hong YM, Cha SH, et al. Epidemiologic features of Kawasaki disease in South Korea: data from nationwide survey, 2009-2011. *Pediatr Infect Dis J* 2014;33:24-7.
9 Lue HC, Chen LR, Lin MT, Chang LY, Wang JK, Lee CY, et al. Epidemiological features of Kawasaki disease in Taiwan, 1976-2007: results of five nationwide questionnaire hospital surveys. *Pediatr Neonatol* 2014;55:92-6.
10 Holman RC, Christensen KY, Belay ED, Steiner CA, Effler PV, Miyamura J, et al. Racial/ethnic differences in the incidence of Kawasaki syndrome among children in Hawaii. *Hawaii Med J* 2010;69:194-7.
11 Moore A, Harnden A, Mayon-White R. Recognising Kawasaki Disease in UK primary care: a descriptive study using the Clinical Practice Research Datalink. *Br J Gen Pract* 2014;64:e477-83.
12 Newburger JW, Takahashi M, Gerber MA, Gewitz MH, Tani LY, Burns JC, et al Diagnosis, treatment, and long-term management of Kawasaki disease: a statement for health professionals from the Committee on Rheumatic Fever, Endocarditis, and Kawasaki Disease, Council on Cardiovascular Disease in the Young, American Heart Association. *Pediatrics* 2004:114:1708-33.
13 Tsuda E, Hamaoka K, Suzuki H, Sakazaki H, Murakami Y, Nakagawa M, et al. A survey of the 3-decade outcome for patients with giant aneurysms caused by Kawasaki disease. *Am Heart J* 2014;167:249-58.
14 Yeom JS, Woo HO, Park JS, Park ES, Seo JH, Youn HS. Kawasaki disease in infants. *Korean J Pediatr* 2013;56:377-82.
15 Benseler SM, McCrindle BW, Silverman ED, Tyrrell PN, Wong J, Yeung RS. Infections and Kawasaki disease: implications for coronary artery outcome. *Pediatrics* 2005;116:e760-6.
16 Wood LE, Tulloh RM. Kawasaki disease in children. *Heart* 2009;95:787-92.
17 Eleftheriou D, Levin M, Shingadia D, Tulloh R, Klein N, Brogan P. Management of Kawasaki disease. *Arch Dis Child* 2014;99:74-83.
18 Yim D, Curtis N, Cheung M, Burgner D.An update on Kawasaki disease II: clinical features, diagnosis, treatment and outcomes. *J Paediatr Child Health* 2013;49:614-23.
19 Tacke CE, Burgner D, Kuipers IM, Kuijpers TW. Management of acute and refractory Kawasaki disease. *Expert Rev Anti Infect Ther* 2012;10:1203-15.
20 Tacke CE, Haverman L, Berk BM, van Rossum MA, Kuipers IM, Grootenhuis MA, et al. Quality of life and behavioral functioning in Dutch children with a history of Kawasaki disease. *J Pediatr* 2012;161:314-9.

Dermatitis herpetiformis

Adam D Jakes, academic foundation doctor[1],
Stephen Bradley, general practitioner trainee[1],
Lynn Donlevy, general practitioner partner[2]

[1]Leeds Teaching Hospitals NHS Trust, Leeds LS9 7TF, UK

[2]Silsden Group Medical Practice, Keighley, UK

Correspondence to: A D Jakes adam.jakes@hyms.ac.uk

Cite this as: *BMJ* 2014;348:g2557

DOI: 10.1136/bmj.g2557

www.bmj.com/content/348/bmj.g2557

A 28 year old woman presented with a raised, red and intensely itchy rash on the extensor surface of her elbows and buttocks, in groups of small blisters. There was no history of trauma, atopy, or recent illness. She had no gastrointestinal symptoms or change in bowel habit and had not lost weight. No major medical or surgical history was noted and she was not taking drugs on a regular basis. Owing to the appearance and location of the rash, together with pruritus, dermatitis herpetiformis was suspected.

What is dermatitis herpetiformis?

Dermatitis herpetiformis is an inflammatory cutaneous condition closely associated with gluten sensitive enteropathy, but the exact mechanism is unknown. It may be the first manifestation of coeliac disease, as at least 75% of patients with dermatitis herpetiformis have some degree of enteropathy, varying from flat mucosa to partial villous atrophy.[1] Gastrointestinal and abdominal symptoms are, however, usually absent.[2] Conversely, only 24% of patients with coeliac disease develop dermatitis herpetiformis.[3] The disease usually presents in young people (ages 15-40 years), is slightly more common in men, and predominately affects white people.[4] The disease follows a chronic-relapsing course.[5] The characteristic pruritic papulovesicular rash is most often evident on the extensor surfaces of elbows (fig 1) and knees, proximal forearms, scalp, and buttocks.[4] Deposition of IgA at the dermal-epidermal junction, following sensitisation by gluten of the gut mucosa, is implicated in the disease and usually holds the key to definitive diagnosis.[6]

How common is dermatitis herpetiformis?

Dermatitis herpetiformis is comparatively rare, with the incidence in northern Europe cited to be between 11.5 and 75.0 per 100 000 population.[7 8 9] Coeliac disease is more common, with a European incidence of approximately 1%.[10] Additionally, coeliac disease is often asymptomatic, with a ratio of symptomatic to asymptomatic disease of 1:5.[4]

The intuition that dermatitis herpetiformis is commonly misdiagnosed by non-dermatologists is widely recognised and often asserted. For example, the National Institutes of Health estimates that "over 95%" of cases are misdiagnosed.[11] Accurate data to quantify the extent of misdiagnosis is, however, lacking. Coeliac disease, on the other hand, is well known for its non-specific presentation and under-diagnosis in primary care.[12]

Why is dermatitis herpetiformis missed?

The vesicular appearance and pruritus of dermatitis herpetiformis means that it is readily mistaken for more common dermatological conditions such as eczema, papular urticaria, and scabies.[2] Uncommon vesiculobullous disorders such as pemphigoid and pemphigus

KEY POINTS

- Dermatitis herpetiformis is a pruritic papulovesicular rash most often found on the extensor surfaces of elbows and knees, proximal forearms, scalp, and buttocks
- Investigations should include serology testing followed by a skin biopsy to confirm the diagnosis
- It is pathognomonic of underlying coeliac disease, and therefore a jejunal biopsy is not required for diagnosis
- Treatment involves a lifelong gluten-free diet, with dapsone used for symptomatic treatment of the rash

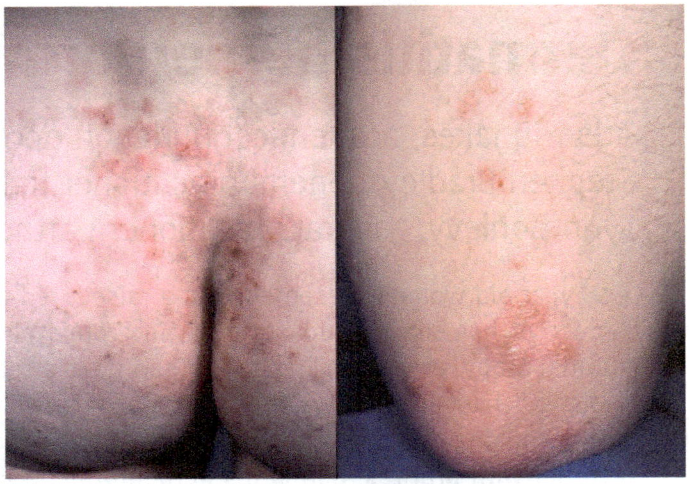

Fig 1 Characteristic pruritic papulovesicular rash of dermatitis herpetiformis, affecting buttocks and elbow. Reprinted with permission of York Hospital and Allan Highet

may also present in a similar pattern. In addition, owing to the pruritic nature of the condition, vesicles are often not seen, and subsequent erosions and excoriations may be mistaken for other diagnoses.

Since symptoms of coeliac disease are present in only around 20% of patients,[2] the possibility of underlying gluten sensitive enteropathy may easily be overlooked.

Why does this matter?

If dermatitis herpetiformis remains undiagnosed, patients may continue to experience intermittent dermatological symptoms and may develop overt coeliac disease, with possible complications of the underlying enteropathy, including osteoporosis, anaemia, and an increased risk of small bowel lymphoma.[13] Adoption of a gluten-free diet may reduce the risk of lymphoma, although evidence is limited and many patients struggle with compliance. Furthermore, misdiagnosis may expose patients to inappropriate treatments, such as corticosteroids in the context of eczema or psoriasis. Recognition of dermatitis herpetiformis may also increase clinical suspicion of associated autoimmune disorders, including Hashimoto's thyroiditis, Sjögren's syndrome, rheumatoid arthritis, sarcoidosis, lupus erythematosus, type 1 diabetes, pernicious anaemia, and Addison's disease.[9]

How is dermatitis herpetiformis diagnosed?

Clinical features

Examination will reveal the distinctive vesicular rash, usually on extensor surfaces. The presence of plaques (psoriasis), interdigital burrows (scabies), or mucosal blistering (pemphigus) should alert the doctor to an alternative diagnosis. Pruritus is often the predominant symptom and can be intense, causing extensive excoriation, which may engender further misidentification for eczema. Ask about fatigue or gastrointestinal symptoms, and check for signs of anaemia. Approximately 10% of patients will have a family history of either coeliac disease or dermatitis herpetiformis.[6]

Investigations

Testing of IgA serology, particularly anti-tissue transglutaminase (sensitivity 98.5%, specificity 98%),[14] will further support the diagnosis of underlying coeliac disease. If serology supports the diagnosis of coeliac disease, useful additional blood tests, including a full blood count, a blood film, haematinics (vitamin B12, folate, ferritin), and urea and electrolytes may highlight deficiencies secondary to intestinal malabsorption. Thyroid function tests are also necessary because of the association of thyroid disease with both coeliac disease and dermatitis herpetiformis.

If the blood tests are indicative of coeliac disease, a referral to secondary care is advocated. Biopsy of unaffected skin in close proximity to an active lesion for direct immunofluorescence is the ideal method of diagnosis and will show granular IgA at the dermal-epidermal junction, with a sensitivity of over 90%[6] (fig 2). Histopathological examination will show an inflammatory infiltrate comprising predominantly neutrophils and eosinophils (fig 2).[7]

Dermatitis herpetiformis, once confirmed, should be considered a cutaneous manifestation of, and pathognomonic for, coeliac disease. This means that duodenal or jejunal biopsies are not considered necessary for further diagnosis.[5] Although the histological findings reflecting gluten sensitive enteropathy will be present in approximately 75% of small bowel biopsies,[1] this is generally only advocated if uncertainty remains as to the diagnosis or if major malabsorption renders obtaining tissue confirmation prudent.[2]

How is dermatitis herpetiformis managed?

The correct diagnosis of dermatitis herpetiformis and subsequently starting a gluten-free diet is the only means to ensure resolution of this condition. Dapsone, an antibacterial agent, can be used for symptomatic relief of the rash, and usually rapidly improves the pruritus. Gradual improvement of symptoms after starting a gluten-free diet and the use of dapsone can take several months. Patients should be counselled about the risks associated with dapsone, which include haemolytic anaemia, agranulocytosis, methaemoglobinaemia, and peripheral neuropathy. Regular full blood counts and directed questions on initiation of dapsone, such as presence of fatigue, numbness, and tingling, and any symptoms suggestive of infection are advised.[2] Once a gluten-free diet has been established, dapsone can be withdrawn slowly.

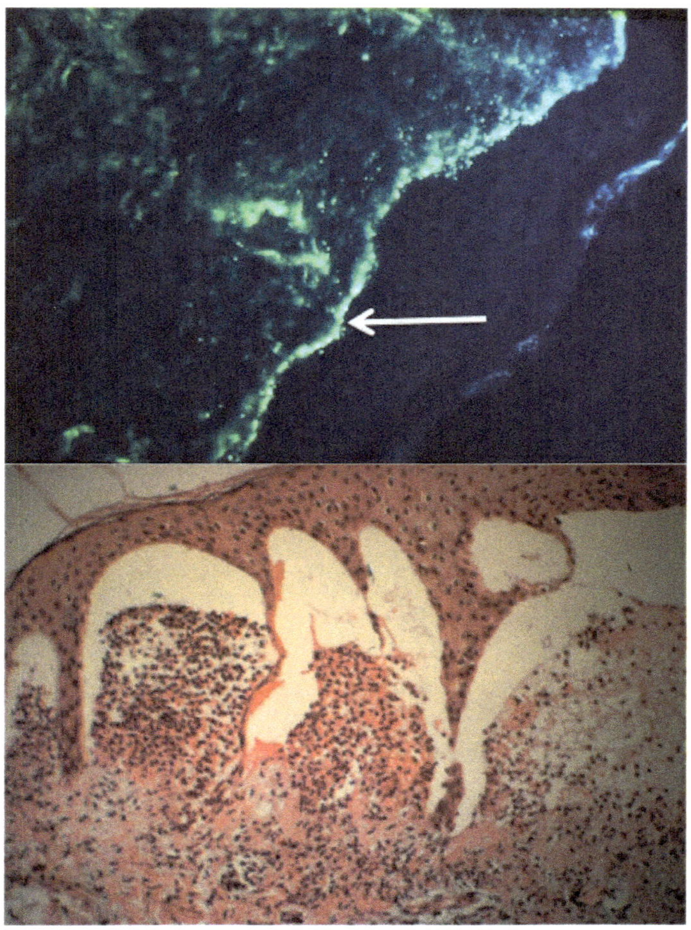

Fig 2 (Top) Direct immunofluorescence showing granular IgA at dermal-epidermal junction (arrow). (Bottom) Histological appearance showing inflammatory infiltrate comprising predominantly neutrophils and eosinophils. Reprinted with permission of York Hospital and Allan Highet

We thank Allan Highet (dermatology consultant, York) and Mark Goodfield (dermatology consultant, Leeds) for their invaluable advice and input.

Contributors: All authors contributed according to ICMJE guidelines. ADJ and SB contributed to planning, drafting, and revising the article and to approval of the final version. LD proposed the article; contributed to revising the article, and is responsible for the overall content as the guarantor.

Competing interests: We have read and understood the BMJ Group policy on declaration of interests and declare: None.

Patient consent not required (patient hypothetical).

1 Collin P, Pukkala E, Reunala T. Malignancy and survival in dermatitis herpetiformis: a comparison with coeliac disease. *Gut* 1996;38:528-30.
2 Herron MD, Zone JJ. Treatment of dermatitis herpetiformis and liner IgA bullous dermatosis. *Dermatol Ther* 2002;15:347-81.
3 Collin P, Reunala T, Rasmussen M, Kyrönpalo S, Pehkonen E, Laippala P, et al. High incidence and prevalence of adult coeliac disease. Augmented diagnostic approach. *Scand J Gastroenterol* 1997;32:1129-33.
4 Fry L. Dermatitis herpetiformis: problems, progress and prospects. *Eur J Dermatol* 2002;12:523-31.
5 Caproni M, Antiga E, Melani L, Fabbri P. Guidelines for the diagnosis and treatment of dermatitis herpetiformis. *J Eur Acad Dermatol Venereol* 2009;23:633-8.
6 Alonso-Llamazares J, Gibson LE, Rogers RS. Clinical, pathologic and immunopathologic features of dermatitis herpetiformis: review of the Mayo Clinic experience. *Int J Dermatol* 2007;46:910-9.
7 Gawkrodger DJ, Blackwell JN, Gilmour HM, Rifkind EA, Heading RC, Barnetson RS. Dermatitis herpetiformis: diagnosis, diet and demography. *Gut* 1984;25:151-7.
8 Salmi TT, Hervonen K, Kautiainen H, Collin P, Reunala T. Prevalence and incidence of dermatitis herpetiformis: a 40-year prospective study from Finland. *Br J Dermatol* 2011;165:354-9.
9 Bolotin D, Petronic-Rosic V. Dermatitis herpetiformis: part I. Epidemiology, pathogenesis, and clinical presentation. *J Am Acad Dermatol* 2011;64:1017-24.
10 Mustalahti K, Catassi C, Reunanen A, Fabiani E, Heier M, McMillan S, et al. The prevalence of celiac disease in Europe: results of a centralized, international mass screening project. *Ann Med* 2010;42:587-95.
11 Services USDoHaH. Celiac Disease Awareness Campaign of the National Institutes of Health. 2013. http://celiac.nih.gov/Dermatitis.aspx.
12 Hin H, Bird G, Fisher P, Mahy N, Jewell D. Coeliac disease in primary care: case finding study. *BMJ* 1999;318:164-7.
13 Grainge MJ, West J, Solaymani-Dodaran M, Card TR, Logan RFA. The long-term risk of malignancy following a diagnosis of coeliac disease or dermatitis herpetiformis: a cohort study. *Aliment Pharmacol Ther* 2012;35:730-9.
14 Alessio Fasano A, Catassi C. Current approaches to diagnosis and treatment of celiac disease: an evolving spectrum. *Gastroenterology* 2001;120:636-51.

More titles in The BMJ Series

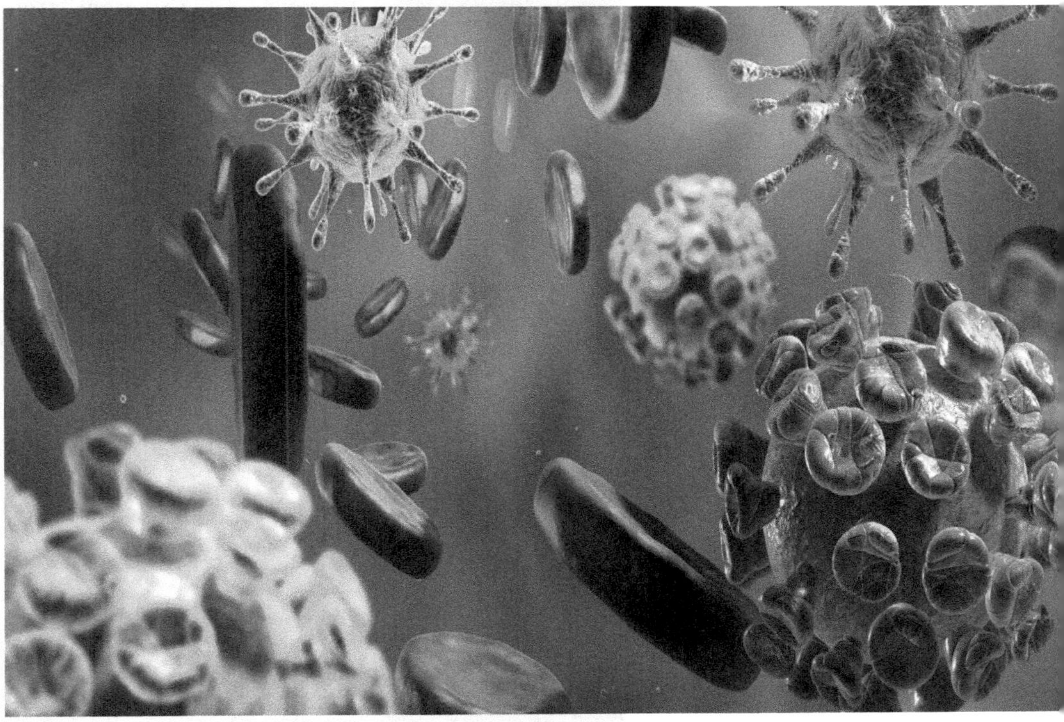

More titles from BPP School of Health

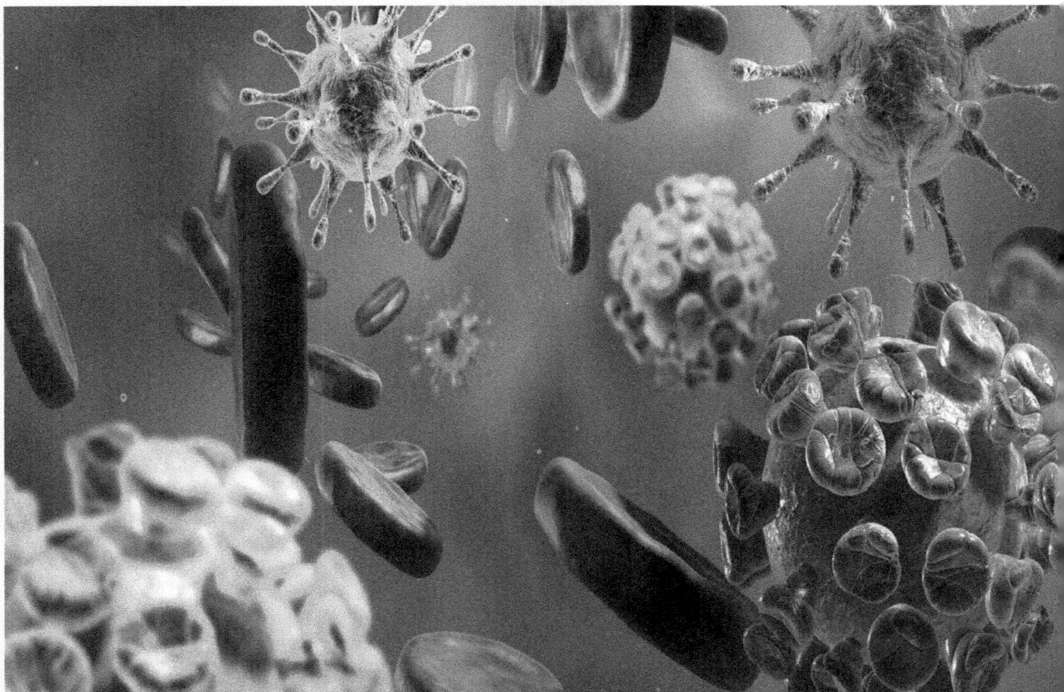

BPP UNIVERSITY SCHOOL OF HEALTH

More titles in The Progressing your Medical Career Series

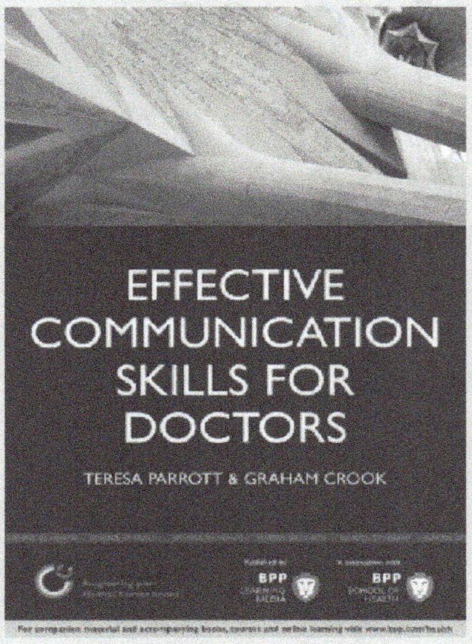

£19.99
September 2011
Paperback
978-1-445379-56-2

Would you like to know how to improve your communication skills? Are you looking for a clearly written book which explores all aspects of effective medical communication?

There is an urgent need to improve doctors' communication skills. Research has shown that poor communication can contribute to patient dissatisfaction, lack of compliance and increased medico-legal problems. Improved communication skills will impact positively on all of these areas.

The last fifteen years have seen unprecedented changes in medicine and the role of doctors. Effective communication skills are vital to these new roles. But communication is not just related to personality. Skills can be learned which can make your communication more effective, and help you to improve your relationships with patients, their families and fellow doctors.

This book shows how to learn those skills and outlines why we all need to communicate more effectively. Healthcare is increasingly a partnership. Change is happening at all levels, from government directives to patient expectations. Communication is a bridge between the wisdom of the past and the vision of the future.

Readers of this book can also gain free access to an online module which upon successful completion can download a certificate for their portfolio of learning/ Revalidation/CPD records.

This easy-to-read guide will help medical students and doctors at all stages of their careers improve their communication within a hospital environment.

BPP UNIVERSITY SCHOOL OF HEALTH

www.bpp.com/medical-series

BPP
UNIVERSITY
SCHOOL OF HEALTH

More titles in The Progressing your Medical Career Series

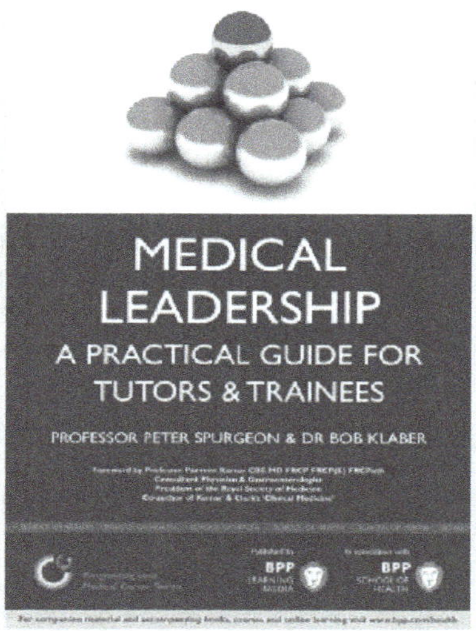

£19.99

November 2011

Paperback

978-1-445379-57-9

Are you a doctor or medical student who wishes to acquire and develop your leadership and management skills? Do you recognise the role and influence of strong leadership and management in modern medicine?

Clinical leadership is something in which all doctors should have an important role in terms of driving forward high quality care for their patients. In this up-to-date guide Peter Spurgeon and Robert Klaber take you through the latest leadership and management thinking, and how this links in with the Medical Leadership Competency Framework. As well as influencing undergraduate curricula and some of the concepts underpinning revalidation, this framework forms the basis of the leadership component of the curricula for all medical specialties, so a practical knowledge of it is essential for all doctors in training.

Using case studies and practical exercises to provide a strong work-based emphasis, this practical guide will enable you to build on your existing experiences to develop your leadership and management skills, and to develop strategies and approaches to improving care for your patients.

This book addresses:

- Why strong leadership and management are crucial to delivering high quality care
- The theory and evidence behind the Medical Leadership Competency Framework
- The practical aspects of leadership learning in a wide range of clinical environments (eg handover, EM, ward etc)
- How Consultants and trainers can best facilitate leadership learning for their trainees and students within the clinical work-place

Whether you are a medical student just starting out on your career, or an established doctor wishing to develop yourself as a clinical leader, this practical, easy-to-use guide will give you the techniques and knowledge you require to excel.

BPP
UNIVERSITY
SCHOOL OF HEALTH

www.bpp.com/medical-series

More titles in The Essential Clinical Handbook Series

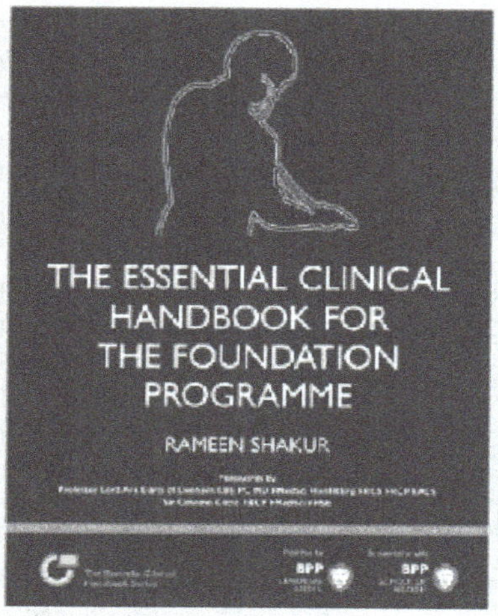

£24.99
October 2011
Paperback
978-1-445381-63-3

Unsure of what clinical competencies you must gain to successfully complete the Foundation Programme? Unclear on how to ensure your ePortfolio is complete to enable your progression to ST training?

This up-to-date clinical handbook is aimed at current foundation doctors and clinical medical students and provides a comprehensive companion to help you in the day-to-day management of patients on the ward. Together with this it is the first handbook to also outline clearly how to gain the core clinical competencies required for successful completion of the Foundation Programme. Written by doctors for doctors this comprehensive handbook explains how to successfully manage all of the common cases you will face during the Foundation Programme and:

- Introduces the Foundation Programme and what is expected of a new doctor especially with the introduction of Modernising Medical Careers
- Illustrates clearly the best way to manage, step-by-step, over 150 commonly encountered clinical diseases, including NICE guidelines to ensure a gold standard of clinical care is achieved
- Describes how to successfully gain the core clinical competencies within Medicine and Surgery including an extensive list of differentials and conditions explained
- Explores the various radiology images you will encounter and how to interpret them
- Tells you how to succeed in the assessment methods used including DOP's, Mini-CEX's and CBD's
- Has step by step diagrammatic guide to doing common clinical procedures competently and safely
- Outlines how to ensure your ePortfolio is maintained properly to ensure successful completion of the Foundation Programme
- Provides tips and advice on how to start preparing now to ensure you are fully prepared and have the competitive edge for your CMT/ST application

The introduction of the e-Portfolio as part of the Foundation Programme has paved the way for foundation doctors to take charge of their own learning and portfolio. Through following the expert guidance laid down in this handbook you will give yourself the best possible chance of progressing successfully through to CMT/ST training.

BPP
UNIVERSITY
SCHOOL OF HEALTH

www.bpp.com/medical-series